Top Articles in Primary Care

John Russell • Neil S. Skolnik
Editors

Top Articles in Primary Care

Springer

Editors
John Russell
Family Medicine
Jefferson Health
Abington, PA, USA

Neil S. Skolnik
Family Medicine
Jefferson Health
Abington, PA, USA

ISBN 978-3-031-25619-6 ISBN 978-3-031-25620-2 (eBook)
https://doi.org/10.1007/978-3-031-25620-2

This Springer imprint is published by the registered company Springer Nature Switzerland AG
The registered company address is: Gewerbestrasse 11, 6330 Cham, Switzerland

John thanks

Elena, Dana, Erin and Paul

for all their love and support

Neil thanks

Alison, Aaron and Ava

who give life meaning, love and purpose

John and Neil would both like to thank

thirty years of residents who inspire our teaching

and who have taught us more than we taught them.

"We stand on the shoulders of giants"

Introduction

The two of us have worked together in the Abington Family Medicine Residency Program for over thirty years. During that time, we have learned more, argued more, joked more, and just had more fun together and with our colleagues than any two people should to be allowed to have over the course of a career. All the time with unending respect for each other's intellect, empathy and humor.

We've taken care of patients and we've taught patient care.

Most relevant to this project, we've shared a love of ideas and the medical literature, and how that literature can be applied to patient care.

All of this is the backstory to this book—a love of the medical literature and a belief that an understanding and appreciation of that literature can enhance our lives as physicians, as well as the lives of our residents, students and patients.

We know that there is no one right answer to what are the top articles in primary care. All of us have our favorites, and inevitably there will be articles here that you will think should not have been included in such esteemed company, and you will have favorites that have been left out. This book will always be a work in progress, it has to be. There is a good chance that a new top article describing a critically important discovery for patients may come out next week. Don't hesitate to let us know if there is an article that you feel should be in here which was not, we'll seriously consider it for our next edition.

We want to take this opportunity to thank a hospital system that supports an academic community hospital family medicine residency and encourages intellectual pursuits, individual growth, innovation and learning.

We also want to thank seven very special individuals—the faculty at Abington Family Medicine—many of whom joined us in this project and with whom we daily share the joys and frustrations of academics, teaching and patient care—Gerald "Trip" Hansen, Mathew Clark, Amy Clouse, Tracey Roesing, Susan Kuchera Fidler, Meera Shah, and Bill Callahan.

Finally, we want to thank our families, who make it all worthwhile and who support us and put up with the sacrifices that a life in academic family medicine entails.

Deepest thanks, from John, to Elena, Dana, Erin, and Paul. Deepest thanks, from Neil, to Alison, Aaron and Ava. We (humbly) feel we have learned so much from each member of our family.

And…ok…thanks to each other.

~~Neil and John~~ John and Neil

Contents

Contributors

Jonathan P. Andrews Jefferson Health, Abington, PA, USA

Chris Azzolino Jefferson Health, Abington, PA, USA

Dimitry Belogorodsky Jefferson Health, Abington, PA, USA

Carrie L. Bender, DO Jefferson Health, Abington, PA, USA

Diana Bonaccorsi Capital Health, Trenton, NJ, USA

Sharon Buchbinder Jefferson Health, Abington, PA, USA

William Callahan Jefferson Health, Abington, PA, USA

Danielle Carcia Capital Health, Trenton, NJ, USA

Sean P. Carnahan UPMC, Pittsburgh, PA, USA

Juliana Carvajal Jefferson Health, Abington, PA, USA

Tricia Cavanaugh Jefferson Health, Abington, PA, USA

Lucy D. Checchio Jefferson Health, Abington, PA, USA

Tina Chuong Jefferson Health, Abington, PA, USA

Mathew Clark Jefferson Health, Abington, PA, USA

Gerard Cleary Jefferson Health, Abington, PA, USA

Sean Cleary Jefferson Health, Abington, PA, USA
Philadelphia College of Osteopathic Medicine, PCOM, Philadelphia, PA, USA

Amy Clouse, MD Jefferson Health, Abington, PA, USA

Robert Danoff Jefferson Health Northeast, Philadelphia, PA, USA

Bryce Eng Jefferson Health, Abington, PA, USA

Susan Kuchera Fidler Jefferson Health, Abington, PA, USA

Alex Scott Fierstein Jefferson Health, Abington, PA, USA

Samantha P. Flanagan, DO Main Line Health, King of Prussia, PA, USA

Katherine Fradeneck Jefferson Health Northeast, Philadelphia, PA, USA

Kevin Franco Jefferson Health, Abington, PA, USA

Evan R. Gooberman Jefferson Health, Abington, PA, USA

Anupriya Grover-Wenk Jefferson Health, Abington, PA, USA

Christian Iversen Jefferson Health, Abington, PA, USA

Angela Kalinowski Jefferson Health, Abington, PA, USA

Morgan Katz Jefferson Health, Abington, PA, USA
Primary Care, ChristianaCare, Newark, USA

Malik Muhammad Uzair Khan Jefferson Health, Abington, PA, USA

Mackenzie Kramer Jefferson Health, Abington, PA, USA

Karen Lazarus Jefferson Health, Abington, PA, USA

Kathleen E. Leary Jefferson Health, Abington, PA, USA

Marie Madden Jefferson Health, Abington, PA, USA

Jeffrey Matthews Jefferson Health, Abington, PA, USA

Thomas McGinley St. Luke's Health, Coaldale, PA, USA

Rameesha Mehreen Jefferson Health, Abington, PA, USA

Merna Mikhail Jefferson Health Northeast, Philadelphia, PA, USA

Hamza Zahid Ullah Muhammadzai Jefferson Health, Abington, PA, USA

Bhasha Mukhopadhyay Jefferson Health Abington, Abington, PA, USA

Ifrah Naeem Jefferson Health, Abington, PA, USA

Marissa Norden Jefferson Health, Abington, PA, USA

Sophie K. Oh Jefferson Health, Abington, PA, USA

Patrick Ottman Jefferson Health, Abington, PA, USA

Gregory Palko Jefferson Health, Abington, PA, USA

Gabriella Petrongolo Jefferson Health, Abington, PA, USA

Binod Poudel Jefferson Health, Abington, PA, USA

Nathaniel Rosal, DO Jefferson Health, Abington, PA, USA

Erin Russell Temple University School of Medicine, Philadelphia, PA, USA
Jefferson Health, Abington, PA, USA

John Russell Jefferson Health, Abington, PA, USA
Family Medicine, Jefferson Health, Philadelphia, PA, USA

Carolyn Sciblo Temple Health Chestnut Hill Family Medicine, Philadelphia, PA, USA

Meera Shah Jefferson Health, Abington, PA, USA

Shreeja Shah Jefferson Health, Abington, PA, USA

Aarisha Shrestha, DO Jefferson Health, Abington, PA, USA

Bridget Smith Jefferson Health, Abington, PA, USA

Rui Song Jefferson Health, Abington, PA, USA

Anne Sprogell Jefferson Health, Abington, PA, USA

Alyssa J. Style Jefferson Health, Abington, PA, USA

Aaron M. Sutton, LCSW, BCD, CAADC Jefferson Health, Abington, PA, USA

Dat Tran Jefferson Health, Abington, PA, USA

Stephanie Tzarnas, MD Jefferson Health, Abington, PA, USA

Dyllan Walter Jefferson Health, Abington, PA, USA

Bree Zeyzus Johns Jefferson Health, Abington, PA, USA

Part I
Behavioral Health

Aaron Sutton

Chapter 1
Treatment Strategies in ADD-1999

Mackenzie Kramer

Background

Attention-deficit hyperactivity disorder (ADHD) is defined by the DSM-V as a persistent pattern of inattention and/or hyperactivity/impulsivity that interferes with functioning and development [1]. ADHD is the most common psychiatric disorder in childhood, affecting 3–5% of school aged children and accounting for 30–50% of child referrals to mental health services [2, 3]. Previous studies have showed the efficacy of short-term treatments of both pharmacotherapy and behavior therapy in treating symptoms of ADHD; however, few controlled studies have followed participants for greater than four months. At the time this study was undertaken, there was a great deal of public concern over the use of stimulants in children with ADHD given the lack of evidence to show that they are effective. This study, the Multimodal Treatment Study of Children With ADHD (MTA), aimed to evaluate pharmacotherapy, behavior therapy, and a combination of the two in a longer-term clinical trial.

The MTA Cooperative Group. A 14-Month Randomized Clinical Trial of Treatment Strategies for Attention-Deficit/Hyperactivity Disorder. Arch Gen Psychiatry. 1999;56(12):1073–1086. doi:10.1001/archpsyc.56.12.1073. https://jamanetwork.com/journals/jamapsychiatry/fullarticle/205525

M. Kramer (✉)
Jefferson Health, Abington, PA, USA
e-mail: Mackenzie.kramer@jefferson.edu

J. Russell, N. S. Skolnik (eds.), *Top Articles in Primary Care*,
https://doi.org/10.1007/978-3-031-25620-2_1

Objective

- To see how long-term medication and behavioral treatments compare with one another when treating children with ADHD, and if there is an additional advantage to using these treatment modalities in combination.
- To evaluate the effectiveness of carefully delivered treatments against routine community care.

Design and Methods

- The study included 579 children, aged 7–9.9 years, with ADHD Combined Type who were randomly assigned to one of the four treatment groups for 14 months.
- Outcomes were measured in distinct groups rated by parents and teachers: primary ADHD symptoms, aggressive and oppositional behavior, internalizing symptoms, for example, anxiety and sadness, social skills, parent–child relationship, and academic achievement.
- Treatment groups included intensive medication management alone, intensive behavioral treatment alone, a combination of both, and routine community care (the control group).
- Behavioral treatment included parent, school, and child components with therapist involvement that gradually reduced over time.
- Medication management was with methylphenidate hydrochloride. If adequate response to methylphenidate was not obtained during titration, alternate medications were titrated openly in the order until a satisfactory response was found: dextroamphetamine, pemoline, imipramine, and, if necessary, others approved by a cross-site panel. Eighty-nine percent completed titration of medication; of these, Sixty-nine percent were assigned to an individually titrated dose of methylphenidate, with average initial doses of 30.5 mg/d. The remaining subjects were openly titrated to dextroamphetamine due to inadequate response to methylphenidate.
- Standard community care involved treatment by community providers. It should be noted that the community care group included many children who received medication and behavioral therapy, since a placebo group with no intervention would have been unethical for this disorder over this period of time.
- Data was analyzed by intent-to-treat random-effects regression procedures over a course of 14 months.

Results

- All 4 groups showed sizable reduction in ADHD symptoms over time, with significant differences between the groups in the degree of improvement.

- Medication management alone, when compared to behavioral treatment alone, showed significant improvements in primary ADHD symptoms, including inattention and hyperactivity-impulsivity, rated by parents and teachers. According to the authors, "Robust differences were found according to 2 different data sources, indicating the superiority of medication management over behavioral treatment for ADHD symptoms."
- When comparing other areas of children's functioning including aggressive and oppositional behavior, peer relations, and academic achievement, medication management alone showed no significant benefit when compared to behavioral treatment alone.
- Children in the combined treatment group and the medication management group showed significant improvement compared to those in the behavioral treatment group as well as the control group. Combined treatment and medication management did not differ significantly across any domain.
- Combined treatment and medication management were superior to community care for parent- and teacher-reported ADHD symptoms. Behavioral treatment showed no significant benefit compared to community care.

Importance

ADHD is the most common psychiatric disorder in childhood and has now been seen to persist into adulthood. This study was the first of its kind to evaluate the differences between pharmacotherapy, behavioral therapy, and a combination of the two in a longer-term clinical trial. While all groups showed a reduction in ADHD symptoms over time, there were important benefits to medication, as well as combined medication and behavioral treatment, with no significant effect of behavioral treatment alone. The MTA updates, which are published approximately every 2 years, give us an insight into more long-term health effects of medication, efficacy, and more research that needs to be done.

Updates

- The MTA was designed and conducted in the early 1990s and underwent eight assessments from the baseline data, published every 2 years.
- In 2007, the MTA published a follow up following 485 of the original 579 children. Among children who continued to take the ADHD medication consistently, the stimulants started to lose effectiveness around three years after treatment was started [2].
- At the 16-year follow up, it was concluded that more than 60% of children, regardless of their medication use, continued to show ADHD symptoms into adulthood [4, 5].

- Multiple studies have shown strong evidence for decreased height associated with prolonged psychostimulant medication taken consistently compared to those who stopped stimulant medication or took it sporadically[5].

Bottom Line

- While all four groups showed improvement over time medication management and combined medication and behavioral therapy were superior to behavioral treatment or community treatment in reducing ADHD symptoms.
- Combined treatment was not better than medication alone for reducing core symptoms of ADHD.
- The authors point out the lack of efficacy of behavioral treatments on the core ADHD symptoms does not mean that behavioral therapy is not important and does not help critical domains of function. ADHD is a chronic disease, the manifestations of which wax and wane over time, often depending upon demands and stressors. Behavioral therapy has values in helping to function optimally given those many issues.
- The original data published in 1999, as well as the extensive follow-up data over the following 16 years, show that an optimal dose of stimulant medication provides children with ADHD an effective way to improve symptoms; however, over time, the medication loses effectiveness.
- The MTA findings challenged the notion that 50% of children with ADHD outgrow the disorder in adulthood. Although intermittent periods of remissions can be expected, approximately 90% of participants in the MTA trial experienced residual ADHD symptoms in young adulthood [6].
- Clinicians must work with their patients to develop an individualized plan for treatment of ADHD and carefully monitor medication prescribed at the correct dose while utilizing other interventions including behavioral therapy.

References

1. Attention-Deficit/Hyperactivity Disorder. Diagnostic and statistical manual of mental disorders: DSM-5. Arlington, VA: American Psychiatric Association; 2013.
2. "The Multimodal Treatment of Attention Deficit Hyperactivity Disorder Study (Mta): Questions and Answers." National Institute of Mental Health, U.S. Department of Health and Human Services, https://www.nimh.nih.gov/funding/clinical research/practical/mta/the-multimodal-treatment-of-attention-deficit-hyperactivity-disorder-study-mtaquestions-and-answers.
3. The MTA Cooperative Group. A 14-month randomized clinical trial of treatment strategies for attention-deficit/hyperactivity disorder. Arch Gen Psychiatry. 1999;56(12):1073–86. https://doi.org/10.1001/archpsyc.56.12.1073.

4. Hechtman L, Swanson JM, Sibley MH, Stehli A, Owens EB, Mitchell JT, Arnold LE, Molina BS, Hinshaw SP, Jensen PS, Abikoff HB, Perez Algorta G, Howard AL, Hoza B, Etcovitch J, Houssais S, Lakes KD, Nichols JQ, MTA Cooperative Group. Functional adult outcomes 16 years after childhood diagnosis of attention-deficit/hyperactivity disorder: MTA results. J Am Acad Child Adolesc Psychiatry. 2016;55(11):945–952.e2. https://doi.org/10.1016/j.jaac.2016.07.774.
5. Editorial: The Continuing Contributions of MTA over Nearly Two Decades to Initial https://acamh.onlinelibrary.wiley.com/doi/full/10.1111/jcpp.12755.
6. Sibley MH, et al. Variable patterns of remission from ADHD in the multimodal treatment study of ADHD. Am J Psychiatr. 2022;179(2):142–51. https://doi.org/10.1176/appi.ajp.2021.21010032.

Chapter 2
Cognitive Behavioral Therapy Versus Medications in Depression-2005

Christian Iversen

Background

Both medications and cognitive therapy had shown efficacy in treatment of depression, including a large study by the Treatment of Depression Collaborative Research Program (TDCRP). This research demonstrated medications were superior to cognitive therapy for severe depression which became the standard of care recommended by the American Psychiatric Association. Prior to this study, there was no randomized, placebo-controlled comparison of medication and cognitive therapy for treatment of moderate to severe depression.

Objective

- To compare efficacy of antidepressant medication and cognitive therapy for treatment of moderate to severe depression.

DeRubeis, R. J., Hollon, S. D., Amsterdam, J. D., Shelton, R. C., Young, P. R., Salomon, R. M., O'Reardon, J. P., Lovett, M. L., Gladis, M. M., Brown, L. L., & Gallop, R. (2005). Cognitive therapy vs medications in the treatment of moderate to severe depression. *Archives of general psychiatry, 62(4)*, 409–416. https://doi.org/10.1001/archpsyc.62.4.409. https://jamanetwork.com/journals/jamapsychiatry/fullarticle/208460

C. Iversen (✉)
Jefferson Health, Abington, PA, USA
e-mail: christian.iversen@jefferson.edu

J. Russell, N. S. Skolnik (eds.), *Top Articles in Primary Care*,
https://doi.org/10.1007/978-3-031-25620-2_2

Design and Methods

- Participants had a diagnosis of major depressive disorder according to DSM IV, were 18–70 years old, spoke English, and could provide informed consent.
- Patients were assessed by the 17-question Hamilton Depression Rating Scale (HDRS) modified to account for both typical and atypical presentations of depression. Patients were required to score 20 or more on two occasions separated by 7 days, and diagnosis was confirmed by a psychiatrist.
- Eligible patients were randomly assigned to medication ($n = 120$), placebo pill ($n = 60$), or cognitive therapy ($n = 60$). Placebo pills were only used for 8 weeks. The medication group was larger to allow additional randomization at the conclusion of this study to assess relapse [1].
- Pharmacology group (paroxetine and placebo pill):
  - Pharmacotherapy sessions conducted by psychiatrists to discuss medications and provide limited supportive counseling. Cognitive therapy techniques were prohibited.
  - Paroxetine doses started at 10–20 mg/day and increased to maximum of 50 mg/day.
  - Patients who failed to respond to paroxetine by 8 weeks were offered additional treatment.
  - Blinding for patients and psychiatrists of the placebo group was broken at 8 weeks, and treatment was offered.
- Cognitive therapy group:
  - Psychologists and a psychiatric nurse practitioner conducted cognitive therapy sessions.
  - Patients were initially treated with 50-min sessions biweekly for 4 weeks with progression to weekly sessions over the subsequent 12 weeks.
- Outcome analysis:
  - The primary endpoint was HDRS reduction at 8 and 16 weeks, with response indicated by a score of 12 or less and stable or decreasing levels at the end of the study.
  - Full remission was defined as HDRS of 7 or less.

Results

- There was nearly equivalent attrition in both medication and cognitive therapy groups. Notably, 5% of the medication group stopped due to side effects or worsening symptoms; approximately 7% stopped therapy for dissatisfaction.
- Paroxetine dose started at 14.0 ± 4.9 mg rising to 37.3 ± 12.4 mg at the end of 16 weeks.

- 47 patients (39%) required augmentation of therapy with lithium, desipramine, venlafaxine, or some combination thereof due to insufficient response on HDRS.
- Both medication and cognitive therapy outperformed placebo to a statistically significant level at 8 weeks. At this point, placebo treatment was discontinued.
- There was no statistically significant difference between medication and cognitive therapy for response rates at 8 or 16 weeks, or for remission at 16 weeks.
- There was evidence that patients with comorbid anxiety responded better to medication, "perhaps because paroxetine [...] has anxiolytic effects".
- There was additional evidence that cognitive therapy at Pennsylvania was more effective than Vanderbilt, "likely related to therapist experience'.

Importance

Similar efficacy was demonstrated for both cognitive therapy and medication for symptomatic improvement and remission of moderate to severe depression in this randomized, placebo-controlled trial. Both treatments were superior to placebo pill. This study provided additional evidence for the therapeutic value of both cognitive therapy and medication management of depression.

Updates

- Patients were followed to assess rates of relapse following completion of the above study [1]. Patients withdrawn from cognitive therapy were less likely to relapse compared with those withdrawn from medication. There was no statistical difference between those withdrawn from therapy and those continuing medication.
- The American Psychiatric Association (APA) recommends second generation antidepressants (SSRI or SNRI), cognitive therapy, or a combination thereof for initial treatment of depression in adults [2]. They additionally suggest cognitive therapy to prevent relapse following remission.

Bottom Line

- Both medication and cognitive therapy provided therapeutic benefit for patients experiencing moderate to severe depression. Relapse was more common following discontinuation of medication compared with therapy. Importantly, therapist experience likely influenced outcomes.

References

1. Hollon S, et al. Prevention of relapse following cognitive therapy vs medications in moderate to severe depression. Arch Gen Psychiatry. 2005;62(4):417–22.
2. American Psychological Association. (2019). Clinical practice guideline for the treatment of depression across three age cohorts. Retrieved from https://www.apa.org/depression-guideline

Chapter 3
Treatment for Major Depressive Disorder (STAR*D)-2008

Aaron M. Sutton

Background

Depression affects approximately 1 in 8 Americans and is the second leading cause of disability-adjusted life years in those 15–44 years old [1]. The majority of individuals with major depressive disorder (MDD) have a chronic or recurrent course and many continue to have symptoms and periods of disability between episodes [2]. Prior to the Sequenced Treatment Alternative to Relieve Depression (STAR*D) trial, there was little evidence in regard to treating patients in real world settings. The majority of previous trials included participants who were recruited through advertisement and who often had few medical or psychiatric comorbidities. In addition, though there had been many trials of the effectiveness of antidepressants in patients with MDD, there was not much evidence about additional anti-depressive treatment that is often needed for the large proportion of patients (up to two-third of patients) who do not respond, or have only a partial response, to first line treatment.

Warden, Diane & Rush, Augustus & Trivedi, Madhukar & Fava, Maurizio & Wisniewski, Stephen. (2008). The STAR*D Project results: A comprehensive review of findings. Current psychiatry reports. 9. 449-59. 10.1007/s11920-007-0061-3 https://link.springer.com/article/10.1007/s11920-007-0061-3

A. M. Sutton (✉)
Jefferson Health, Abington, PA, USA
e-mail: aaron.sutton@jefferson.edu

J. Russell, N. S. Skolnik (eds.), *Top Articles in Primary Care*,
https://doi.org/10.1007/978-3-031-25620-2_3

Objective

The STAR*D trial aimed to develop treatment strategies that would improve clinical outcomes in patients with treatment resistant depression, who were experiencing a major depressive episode. Specifically, the trial focused on how to initiate treatment and what the next steps in treatment would be, should participants not reach remission or cannot tolerate the treatment.

Design and Methods

- Over a 7-year period, 4041 outpatients between 18 and 75 years of age were enrolled from 41 clinical sites across the country; 2876 were eligible and began level 1. Level 2 results included 1439, level 3 included 377, and level 4 included 142.
- In level 1, participants were given citalopram (Celexa) for 12–14 weeks. If patients became symptom free, they could move to a 12-month follow-up program in which Celexa was continued and patients were monitored. If participants could not tolerate Celexa, or did not become symptom free, they moved to level 2.
- Participants in level 2 had the option of switching medication or adding medication to Celexa. Those who switched were randomly assigned either sertraline (Zoloft), bupropion-SR (Wellbutrin), or Venlafaxine XR (Effexor). If augmenting, participants were randomly assigned bupropion-SR (Wellbutrin) or buspirone to continue with Celexa. Participants also had the option of adding on or switching to cognitive therapy. As in level 1, if participants became symptom free, they would continue with treatment and those who did not or could not tolerate treatment moved to level 3.
- Level 3, like level 2, allowed participants the opportunity to switch or augment. If switching, participants were randomly assigned either mirtazapine (Remeron) or nortriptyline (Aventyl or Pamelor) for up to 14 weeks. In the augmentation group, participants were randomly assigned to lithium or triiodothyronine (T3). As in previous levels, if participants became symptom free, they would be monitored and those who did not or could not tolerate medications proceeded to level 4.
- Participants in level 4 were taken off any previous medications and randomly switched to either the monoamine oxidase inhibitor (MAOI) tranylcypromine (Parnate) or the combination of venlafaxine extended release (Effexor XR) with mirtazapine (Remeron).

Results

- The majority of clinical trials for depression use a measure of success called "response," which means that symptoms have decreased to at least half of what they were when starting a trial. However, the STAR*D trial uses the measure of remission, meaning that participants were symptom free, however notates response as well.
- In level 1, remission rates were between 28 and 33% with further response rate between 10 and 15% depending on what measurement was used for assessment, either the Hamilton Depression Rating Scale (HDRS) or Quick Inventory for Depression Screening (QIDS).
- At level 2, patients who did not have a full response to citalopram were switched to either bupropion-SR, sertraline, and venlafaxine-XR. About one-fourth of patients who had a medication switch experienced a remission, and remission rates for bupropion-SR, sertraline, and venlafaxine-XR were similar.
- At level 2 patients could choose augmentation with bupropion-SR or buspirone. Patients treated with bupropion-SR showed greater symptom improvement, lower symptom severity, and fewer dropouts due to intolerance.
- Cognitive therapy had equal efficacy when used as a level 2 augmentation strategy as when medication was used to augment citalopram. When used as "switch therapy," i.e., when patients stopped their level 1 citalopram therapy and switched to either a different medicine or cognitive therapy, a fourth of patients had equal efficacy to switching medications, with approximately a fourth of patients in both groups showing a response.
- Level 3 remission rates varied between switching to mirtazapine (12%) and augmentation with triiodothyronine or T3 (25%). Again, there were no statistically significant differences in medications used.
- In level 4, the remission rate from switching to tranylcypromine was 7%, while the combination of venlafaxine extended release (Effexor XR) with mirtazapine (Remeron) was 14%.

Importance

With an estimated 16 million Americans experiencing a depressive episode in a given year, family physicians are on the front line of providing care. Currently, general practitioners prescribe about 60% of all psychotropic medications with family medicine physicians being a majority in that group [3]. It is important to understand all treatment options including how to initiate treatment, augmenting treatment, providing options and rationale for psychotherapy, and discussing expectations for treatment with patients.

Updates

- Multiple articles have been published since the results of STAR*D were published asking for further evaluation of results based on biases. Potential detriments to the study include "treat to remission method," overstated estimates of remission, acknowledgement of participants that dropped out through step 3, and an assumption that those who dropped out could be included in the group that was successfully treated [4].

Bottom Line

- Primary care physicians can effectively treat depression in a primary care "real world" setting. Many patients who do not achieve remission or response after a few weeks typically do so after 14 weeks. If initial treatment with an SSRI does not lead to full remission, the evidence supports additional therapeutic approaches. The therapeutic approach can be effective in leading to remission either by switching to a different anti-depressant, or by augmenting the initial treatment with bupropion-SR. Cognitive therapy had efficacy equal to medication as second level therapy either by switching to cognitive therapy or augmenting the existent medication with cognitive therapy.

References

1. Indian J Psychol Med. 2010;32(1):1–2.
2. Bains N, Abdijadid S. Major Depressive Disorder. [Updated 2022 Jun 1]. In: StatPearls [Internet]. Treasure Island (FL): StatPearls Publishing; 2022.
3. Barkil-Oteo A. Collaborative care for depression in primary care: how psychiatry could "troubleshoot" current treatments and practices. Yale J Biol Med. 2013;86(2):139–46. PMID: 23766735; PMCID: PMC3670434.
4. Pigott HE. The STAR*D Trial: It Is Time to Reexamine the Clinical Beliefs That Guide the Treatment of Major Depression. Can J Psychiatry. 2015;60(1):9–13. https://doi.org/10.1177/070674371506000104. PMID: 25886544; PMCID: PMC4314062.

Chapter 4
Depression Screening Questions-2017

Carolyn Sciblo

Background

Depression is a common disorder in older adults with a prevalence of 10–20%. It is even more common among those with illnesses and/or living in residential facilities. The United States Preventative Services Task Force recommends screening for depression in older adults. However, depressive symptoms can be similar to symptoms of physical illness. Older adults may complain of physical discomfort rather than depressive symptoms, making depression difficult to diagnose in this population.

Objective

1. Evaluate the accuracy of the two-question screen for older adults and compare it with other screening tools for depression (see Table 4.1).

Reference: Tsoi KKF, Chan JYC, Hirai HW, et al. Comparison of diagnostic performance of Two-Question Screen and 15 depression screening instruments for older adults: systematic review and meta-analysis. BJP 2017; 210:255-260.
Hyperlink PDF: https://www.cambridge.org/core/services/aop-cambridge-core/content/view/480AB1EC2A48754582F77456C2D7A1D0/S0007125000281099a.pdf/comparison_of_diagnostic_performance_of_twoquestion_screen_and_15_depression_screening_instruments_for_older_adults_systematic_review_and_metaanalysis.pdf

---

C. Sciblo (✉)
Temple Health Chestnut Hill Family Medicine, Philadelphia, PA, USA

J. Russell, N. S. Skolnik (eds.), *Top Articles in Primary Care*,
https://doi.org/10.1007/978-3-031-25620-2_4

Table 4.1 Two-question screen for depression

Have you been troubled by feeling down, depressed or hopeless?	During the past month, have you often been bothered by having little interest or pleasure in doing things?

Design and Methods

1. This systematic review assessed 132 studies evaluating 16 depression screening instruments and included 143 cohorts from more than 30 countries.
2. Studies included older adults with mean or median age of 60 or older, used standard diagnostic criteria to diagnose depression (such as DSM), and reported the number of participants with depression as well as the accuracy of screening instruments.
3. Main outcome was the accuracy of screening tools to diagnose depression in older adults.
4. Subgroup analysis was also performed to assess the screening tools in nursing home, specialist clinic settings, and community settings.

Results

1. Of the 16 tools evaluated, 13 were self-rating scales, two were clinician-rated scales, and one was rated by the clinician and informant.
2. All but one tool, the one-question screen, showed good diagnostic accuracy.
3. Seven cohorts from six studies reported on the diagnostic accuracy of the two-question screen, and all used one as the cut-off value for the two-question screen (one) compared to varying cut-off values for other tools.
4. The two-question screen also had good diagnostic accuracy in the subgroup analysis.

Importance

Depression is a common issue in older adults that can further complicate concurrent problems. Depression in older adults is associated with increased risk of death and disability, as well as an increased risk of dementia [1]. Rates of major depressive disorder rise with increasing medical morbidity [2]. Thus, medically complex older adults are more likely to have depression. Screening for depression is an important aspect of geriatric care, but clinicians need to be efficient when caring for these complex patients. The two-question screen is a self-rating scale that is completed by the patient answering two yes/no questions. This study showed that the two-question screen had similar, or superior accuracy when compared to fifteen other screening tools. Additionally, it is simple and quick to incorporate into clinical practice.

Bottom Line

Depression screening is important in the care of older adults, and the two-question screen is an accurate tool that can be easily and quickly performed in practice.

References

1. Rodda J, Walker Z, Carter J. Depression in older adults. BMJ. 2011;343:d5219.
2. Taylor WD. Depression in the elderly. N Engl J Med. 2014;371:1228–36.

Part II
Cardiovascular Disease

Neil Skolnik

Chapter 5
Pre-operative Clearance (Goldman Criteria)-1977

Shreeja Shah

Background

Major Adverse Cardiac Events (MACEs) are common in patients undergoing noncardiac surgeries. Until 1977, the most widely used technique for perioperative assessment of surgical risk was from the Dripps-American Surgical Association, which only predicted perioperative noncardiac complications. Pre-existing data that suggested correlation of recent preoperative myocardial infarction and cardiac disease with overall surgery and cardiac risk were only limited to univariate analysis. This study attempted to make a multifactorial approach to estimate cardiac risk in noncardiac surgical procedures.

Objective

- To determine which preoperative factors affect the development of cardiac complications after major noncardiac operations.

Lee Goldman, Debra L. Caldera, Samuel R. Nussbaum, et al. The New England Journal of Medicine. Massachusetts Medical Society. Oct 20, 1977. https://www.nejm.org/doi/full/10.1056/nejm197710202971601

S. Shah (✉)
Jefferson Health, Abington, PA, USA
e-mail: Shreeja.Shah@jefferson.edu

J. Russell, N. S. Skolnik (eds.), *Top Articles in Primary Care*,
https://doi.org/10.1007/978-3-031-25620-2_5

Design and Methods

- This is a prospective study which included 1001 patients over 40 years of age operated on by general surgery, orthopedic surgery, and urology services at Massachusetts General Hospital, or by 11 co-operating private surgeons between October 1975 and April 1976.
- Preoperative factors were defined and recorded by taking history and detailed physical examination, obtaining pertinent laboratory data, electrocardiogram, and chest X-ray prior to surgery. Occasional cases of emergency late-night operations were an exception.
- Prospectively, all cardiac complications that developed before hospital discharge were recorded.
- Primary outcome was death from cardiac cause or any of three major complications—myocardial infarction, pulmonary edema, ventricular tachycardia. Other complications were considered minor.
- Multivariate linear discriminant analysis was performed to determine correlation of the preoperative factors with primary outcome.

Results

- 19 patients died postoperatively due to cardiac causes, 18 suffered from intra/postoperative myocardial infarction, 36 had pulmonary edema, and 12 had documented ventricular tachycardia.
- Nine preoperative factors were determined to have statistically significant independent correlations with cardiac outcome (Table 5.1).
- For clinical purposes, discriminant-function coefficients were used to calculate "point" value for the factor associated and four risk categories were defined: class I (points 0–5), class II (points 6–12), class III (points 13–25), and class IV (>26 points).
- No or only minor complication occurred in: 99% of class I patients, 93% of class II, 86% of class III, and 22% of class IV patients. Life threatening complications were: 0.7% in class I, 5% in class II, 11% in class III and 22% in class IV. Cardiac deaths were: 0.2% in class I, 2% in class II and III, and 56% in class IV.
- It was also noted that Dripps-American Surgical Association class did not add a statistically significant increment in classification power to that of the nine-factor index.

Table 5.1 Pre-operative factors

Perioperative factors	Points
1. History	
Age >70	5
MI in previous 6 mo	10
2. Physical exam	
a. S3 gallop or JVD	11
b. Important VAS	3
3. EKG	
a. Rhythm other than sinus or PACs on Preop EKG	7
b. >5 PVC/min any time before operation	7
4. General status	
$PO_2 < 60$ or $PCO_2 > 50$ mmHg, $K < 3.0$ or $HCO_3 < 20$ meq/l, BUN > 50 or Cr > 3.0 mg/dl, abnormal SGOT, signs of chronic liver disease or patient bed ridden from noncardiac causes	3
5. Operation	
a. Intraperitoneal, intrathoracic, or aortic operation	3
b. Emergency operation	4

Importance

This study helped in substantiating correlation of postoperative cardiac complications with recent preoperative myocardial infarction and separated these patients into high-risk and low-risk subgroups by applying multifactorial index. It also confirmed the correlation of cardiac complications with emergency operations. Premature ventricular contractions had not been reported previously as a factor for perioperative cardiac complications which was established in this study.

The cardiac risk index derived from this study helped in estimating additional cardiac risk to surgical risk and therefore estimate overall morbidity and mortality. It also recommended different approaches based on risk class. It led to routine preoperative cardiac consultation for class III and recommended only truly life-saving procedures be performed on class IV patients. This risk calculation was the first of its kind and paved a pathway for future cardiac risk stratification.

Updates

- In 1999, Revised Cardiac Risk Index (RCRI) was developed by Lee et al. that evaluates six independent variables (type of surgery, ischemic heart disease, congestive heart failure, cerebrovascular disease, diabetes mellitus, and renal function) for cardiac outcome. In 2009 and 2014, the European Society of Cardiology (ESC) and European Society of Anesthesiology (ESA) included this index in their preoperative cardiac risk assessment. It was also recommended by American College of Cardiology (ACC) and American Heart Association (AHA) in their 2014 guidelines [1, 2].
- In 2007, the American College of Surgeons National Surgical Quality Improvement Program (NSQIP) database risk model was developed. ACS-NSQIP or American College of Surgeons Surgical Risk Calculator (ACS-SRC) was based on this model which included 21 preoperative factors. While more comprehensive, it is cumbersome and requires an online tool [3].
- In 2011, Gupta risk calculator was developed by Gupta et al. to calculate Myocardial Infarction and Cardiac Arrest (MICA) based on five preoperative predictors. The recent ESC/ESA guidelines recommend its use in addition to RCRI (Class I recommendation, level of evidence B) [4].

Bottom Line

- Cardiac risk index derived from this study not only helped in risk stratification but also helped in facilitating decision-making to improve patient outcome. It opened an arena for existing risk indices and has helped in developing safer perioperative strategies for cardiac optimization.

References

1. Lee TH, Marcantonio ER, Mangione CM, Thomas EJ, Polanczyk CA, Cook EF, Sugarbaker DJ, Donaldson MC, Poss R, Ho KK, Ludwig LE, Pedan A, Goldman L. Derivation and prospective validation of a simple index for prediction of cardiac risk of major noncardiac surgery. Circulation. 1999;100(10):1043–9. https://doi.org/10.1161/01.cir.100.10.1043. PMID: 10477528.
2. Kristensen SD, Knuuti J, Saraste A, Anker S, Bøtker HE, Hert SD, Ford I, Gonzalez-Juanatey JR, Gorenek B, Heyndrickx GR, Hoeft A, Huber K, Iung B, Kjeldsen KP, Longrois D, Lüscher TF, Pierard L, Pocock S, Price S, Roffi M, Sirnes PA, Sousa-Uva M, Voudris V, Funck-Brentano C, Authors/Task Force Members. 2014 ESC/ESA guidelines on non-cardiac surgery: cardiovascular assessment and management: the Joint Task Force on non-cardiac surgery: cardiovascular assessment and management of the European Society of Cardiology (ESC) and the European Society of Anaesthesiology (ESA). Eur Heart J. 2014;35(35):2383–431. https://doi.org/10.1093/eurheartj/ehu282. Epub 2014 Aug 1. PMID: 25086026.

3. Bilimoria KY, Liu Y, Paruch JL, Zhou L, Kmiecik TE, Ko CY, Cohen ME. Development and evaluation of the universal ACS NSQIP surgical risk calculator: a decision aid and informed consent tool for patients and surgeons. J Am Coll Surg. 2013;217(5):833–42. https://doi.org/10.1016/j.jamcollsurg.2013.07.385. Epub 2013 Sep 18. PMID: 24055383; PMCID: PMC3805776.
4. Gupta PK, Gupta H, Sundaram A, Kaushik M, Fang X, Miller WJ, Esterbrooks DJ, Hunter CB, Pipinos II, Johanning JM, Lynch TG, Forse RA, Mohiuddin SM, Mooss AN. Development and validation of a risk calculator for prediction of cardiac risk after surgery. Circulation. 2011;124(4):381–7. https://doi.org/10.1161/CIRCULATIONAHA.110.015701. Epub 2011 Jul 5. PMID: 21730309.

Chapter 6
Thrombolysis in Acute Strokes (ECASS-II)-1998

Patrick Ottman

Background

Cerebral vascular accidents (CVA) (strokes) affect 795,000 people in the USA annually which equates to a stroke every 40 seconds [1]. Of these strokes, 87% are ischemic in nature which means they occur from blood vessel blockages [1]. These blood vessel blockages are sometimes amendable to therapy with a clot dissolver called tissue plasminogen activator (TPA) [1]. The ECASS II trial was one of the first trials to review the safety and efficacy of alteplase (recombinant TPA) which to this day is still one of the first line therapies for ischemic CVA.

Objective

- Assess the safety and efficacy of alteplase (recombinant TPA) at a dose of 0.9 mg/kg bodyweight within 6 h of stroke onset.

Hacke, W., Kaste, M., Fieschi, C., von Kummer, R., Davalos, A., Meier, D., Larrue, V., Bluhmki, E., Davis, S., Donnan, G., Schneider, D., Diez-Tejedor, E., & Trouillas, P. Randomised double-blind placebo-controlled trial of thrombolytic therapy with intravenous alteplase in acute ischaemic stroke (ECASS II). Second European-Australasian Acute Stroke Study Investigators. Lancet (London, England), 1998;352(9136):1245–51. https://doi.org/10.1016/s0140-6736(98)08020-9
Hyperlink to PDF: https://pubmed.ncbi.nlm.nih.gov/9788453/

P. Ottman (✉)
Jefferson Health, Abington, PA, USA
e-mail: Patrick.ottman@jefferson.edu

J. Russell, N. S. Skolnik (eds.), *Top Articles in Primary Care*,
https://doi.org/10.1007/978-3-031-25620-2_6

Design and Methods

- Trial enrolled 800 patients from Europe, Australia, and New Zealand aged 18–80 years old who were:
  - Diagnosed with a moderate or severe ischemic hemispheric stroke
  - Could be treated within 6 h of onset
  - Showed no/only minor early signs of infarction on their initial head CT
  - Could follow-up in 90 days
- Randomized, double blinded placebo-controlled trial grouped by time of onset (0–3 h or 3–6 h)
- Primary endpoint: Modified Rankin scale (mRS) at 90 days with scores 0–1 (favorable) and score 2–6 (unfavorable)
- Analyses: Intention to treat

Results

- Results found a benefit of alteplase over placebo; however, it was not statistically significant.
  - Previous trials though had found a statistically significant improved functional outcome when alteplase was compared to placebo.
  - Post-hoc analysis using the mRS categorized based on individual scores (mRS score 0, 1 or 2) did find a favorable difference (using Fisher's exact test) for alteplase but this was not the pre-defined primary end point.
- No significant differences in the primary and secondary outcomes were found between patients treated at 0–3 h or 3–6 h although there were only a small number of patients in the 0–3 h group.
- No significant difference in patient death between alteplase and placebo.
- Increased risk of symptomatic intracranial hemorrhage with alteplase compared to placebo.

Importance

ECASS II was one of the first trials to review alteplase's safety and efficacy which is significant as alteplase is still one of the first line therapies for ischemic CVA. Alteplase was examined by two trials prior to this study [2, 3]. Approval for alteplase in the USA was granted after the National Institute of Neurological Disorders and Stroke (NINDS) trial found better functional outcomes without increased mortality when treated within 3 h of symptoms at a dose of 0.9 mg/kg bodyweight [2]. The second trial was ECASS I which examined alteplase at 1.1 mg/kg bodyweight within 6 h of symptom onset and found a favorable significant difference in functional outcome when compared to placebo but mortality was increased [3]. After these results, ECASS II was created to evaluate the lower dose of alteplase used in NINDS to see if the increased mortality from ECASS I could be minimized but still achieve favorable outcomes with alteplase given within 6 h of symptom onset [2, 3]. This study has helped alteplase remain one of the leading therapies of ischemic CVA now indicated up to 4.5 h after symptom onset.

Updates

To help address ECASS II's findings of no statistical difference in benefit of alteplase over placebo during a 6 h timeline but to extend the 3 h timeline used in NINDS, ECASS III was created using the same dose of alteplase (0.9 mg/kg bodyweight) with a timeline for administration of 3–4.5 h after onset of symptoms [2, 4]. ECASS III, with alteplase given up to 4.5 h after symptoms, found a significant improvement in patient outcomes (defined as disability at 90 days based on the mRS as above) without an increase in mortality or a further increase in intracranial hemorrhage compared to alteplase given within 3 h in NINDS [2, 4]. The combination of these findings has formed the backbone of current therapy with TPA given 3–4.5 h after the onset of symptoms.

Bottom Line

- While ECASS II did not show a statistical benefit of alteplase over placebo there was a favorable difference using Fisher's exact test when not using the predefined primary end point and there was no increased mortality when alteplase was given within 6 h after symptom onset

References

1. Virani SS, Alonso A, Benjamin EJ, Bittencourt MS, et al. Heart disease and stroke statistics-2020 update: A report from the American Heart Association. Circulation. 2020;141(9):e139–596. https://doi.org/10.1161/CIR.0000000000000757.
2. National Institute of Neurological Disorders and Stroke rt-PA Stroke Study Group. Tissue plasminogen activator for acute ischemic stroke. N Engl J Med. 1995;333(24):1581–7. https://doi.org/10.1056/NEJM199512143332401.
3. Hacke W, Kaste M, Fieschi C, Toni D, Lesaffre E, von Kummer R, Boysen G, Bluhmki E, Höxter G, Mahagne MH. Intravenous thrombolysis with recombinant tissue plasmino-

gen activator for acute hemispheric stroke. The European Cooperative Acute Stroke Study (ECASS). JAMA. 1995;274(13):1017–25. PMID: 7563451.

4. Hacke W, Kaste M, Bluhmki E, Brozman M, Dávalos A, Guidetti D, Larrue V, Lees KR, Medeghri Z, Machnig T, Schneider D, von Kummer R, Wahlgren N, Toni D, Investigators ECASS. Thrombolysis with alteplase 3 to 4.5 hours after acute ischemic stroke. N Engl J Med. 2008;359(13):1317–29. https://doi.org/10.1056/NEJMoa0804656. PMID: 18815396.

Chapter 7
Rate Versus Rhythm Control in Atrial Fibrillation (AFFIRM)-2002

Samantha P. Flanagan

Background

Atrial fibrillation (Afib) is a common condition, affecting an estimated 2.7–6.1 million people in the USA [1]. Atrial fibrillation more commonly affects individuals over the age of 65. Afib increases an individual's stroke risk by four to five times [2]. The AFFIRM trial was the first and largest trial to compare rate control vs. rhythm control for the management of Afib.

Objective

- To compare the two most commonly used strategies for the management of atrial fibrillation, rate control and rhythm control.

Design and Methods

- The study included just over 4000 patients aged 65 or greater in a randomized multi-center comparison with the primary endpoint of mortality.

Wyse DG, Waldo AL, DiMarco JP, et al. A comparison of rate control and rhythm control in patients with atrial fibrillation. N Engl J Med 2002; 347: 1825.
Article PDF: https://www.ahajournals.org/doi/pdf/10.1161/01.CIR.0000121736.16643.11

S. P. Flanagan (✉)
Main Line Health, King of Prussia, PA, USA

J. Russell, N. S. Skolnik (eds.), *Top Articles in Primary Care*,
https://doi.org/10.1007/978-3-031-25620-2_7

- The study did not compare specific medications head-to-head but rather allowed physicians to tailor treatment to patients.
  - Rhythm-control medications: amiodarone, disopyramide, flecainide, moricizine, procainamide, propafenone, quinidine, sotalol, and dofetilide.
  - Rate-control medications: beta-blockers, calcium-channel blockers, and digoxin.
- Anticoagulation using warfarin was mandated with a goal INR of 2.0–3.0, but could be stopped in the rhythm-control group if sinus rhythm was maintained for at least 4 weeks.
- Data was evaluated with an intention-to-treat analysis.

Results

- More deaths occurred in the rhythm-control group than the rate-control group; however, mortality differences between the two groups were not statistically significant.
- Stroke occurred at approximately 1% per year in both groups. Most strokes occurred in patients who had stopped taking warfarin and those with subtherapeutic INRs.
- Patients in the rhythm-control group were significantly more likely to be hospitalized and have adverse drug reactions than those in the rate-control group. Additionally, torsade de pointes, bradycardia arrest, and hospitalization occurred more often in the rhythm-control group than in the rate-control group.

Importance

The AFFIRM trial played a major role in determining strategies for the management of atrial fibrillation. Prior to the study, most physicians primarily attempted rhythm control in patients with Afib and used rate control as a back-up means to management. After this trial, either modality could be used as the initial treatment for Afib.

It is also important to note that anticoagulation played an important role in the study as results showed that patients who had stopped anticoagulation or who had subtherapeutic INRs were more likely to suffer from stroke regardless of whether they were rate or rhythm controlled. In 2002, when AFFIRM was published the only oral anticoagulant available was warfarin. Today there are several direct oral anticoagulants that can be used to anticoagulate patients with non-valvular Afib.

Updates

- A follow-up report from the AFFIRM Investigators issued several years after the initial article looked at the same data using an "on-treatment" analysis rather than an intention-to-treat analysis. This review concluded that sinus rhythm was an important determinant of survival, suggesting that the adverse effects of these medications nullify the added benefits of maintaining sinus rhythm [3].
- RACE II (*Lenient versus Strict Rate Control in Patients with Atrial Fibrillation)* compared strict (<80 beats/min) to lenient (<110 beats/min) rate control and found that both were equally effective at preventing adverse cardiac events [4].
- EAST-AFNET 4 (*Early Rhythm-Control Therapy in Patients with Atrial Fibrillation*) was published in the New England Journal in October 2020 and investigated rhythm vs. rate control in 2789 patients with early Afib. Early rhythm-control was defined as diagnosis less than 1 year before enrollment. The initial primary end point was a composite of death from cardiovascular causes, stroke, or hospitalization with worsening of heart failure or acute coronary syndrome. Rhythm control included treatment with antiarrhythmic drugs or catheter ablation. This study showed that early rhythm-control was associated with lower risk of adverse cardiovascular outcomes compared with usual care in those patients with early Afib and cardiovascular conditions [5].

Bottom Line

- The AFFIRM trial demonstrated that rate control and rhythm control are equal in regard to mortality benefit, but rate-control medications are safer to use compared to rhythm-control medications. Patients with atrial fibrillation should be anticoagulated. Subsequent trials suggest that early rhythm control with selective use of catheter ablation may be the optimal approach for new onset Afib.

References

1. January CT, Wann LS, Alpert JS, Calkins H, Cigarroa JE, Cleveland JC Jr, et al. 2014 AHA/ACC/HRS guideline for the management of patients with atrial fibrillation. J Am Coll Cardiol. 2014;64(21):2246–80.
2. Mozaffarian D, Benjamin EJ, Go AS, Arnett DK, Blaha MJ, Cushman M, et al. Heart disease and stroke statistics—2015 update: a report from the American Heart Association. Circulation. 2015;131:e29–e322.

3. Corley SD, Epstein AE, DiMarco JP, Domansk MJ, Geller N, Greene HL, Wyse DG. Relationships between sinus rhythm, treatment, and survival in the atrial fibrillation follow-up investigation of rhythm management (AFFIRM) study. Circulation. 2004;109(12):1509–13. https://doi.org/10.1161/01.cir.0000121736.16643.11.
4. Gelder IC, Groenveld HF, Crijns HJ, Tuininga YS, Tijssen JG, Alings AM, Berg MP. Lenient versus strict rate control in patients with atrial fibrillation. N Engl J Med. 2010;362(15):1363–73. https://doi.org/10.1056/nejmoa1001337.
5. Kirchof P, Camm AJ, Goette A, Brandes A, et al. Early rhythm-control therapy in patients with atrial fibrillation. N Engl J Med. 383(14):1305–16. https://doi.org/10.1056/NEJMoa2019422.

Chapter 8
Defibrillators in Low-Ejection Fraction Patients (MADIT-II)-2002

Binod Poudel

Background

Sudden cardiac death due to ventricular arrhythmias can occur in patients with a history of myocardial infarction and reduced left ventricular ejection fraction (LVEF).

Objective

- To evaluate the potential survival benefit of implantable defibrillators in patients with a history of myocardial infarction (MI) and severe left ventricular dysfunction.

Design and Methods

- This was a randomized controlled trial involving 1232 participants.
- All participants were at least 21 years of age, had a myocardial infarction at least one month prior, and had a LVEF of 30% or less.

Moss, A. J., Zareba, W, et al. (2002). Prophylactic implantation of a defibrillator in patients with myocardial infarction and reduced ejection fraction. The New England Journal of Medicine, 346(12), 877–883. https://www.nejm.org/doi/full/10.1056/nejmoa013474

B. Poudel (✉)
Jefferson Health, Abington, PA, USA
e-mail: Binod.Poudel@jefferson.edu

J. Russell, N. S. Skolnik (eds.), *Top Articles in Primary Care*,
https://doi.org/10.1007/978-3-031-25620-2_8

- Participants were not required to undergo electrophysiologic (EP) studies for risk stratification.
- Exclusion criteria included recent myocardial infarction within the last month, coronary revascularization in the preceding three months, or having an FDA-approved indication for defibrillator.
- Participants were randomly assigned to receive either conventional medical therapy with an implantable defibrillator (treatment group) or conventional medical therapy alone (control group). Conventional medical therapy included the use of ACEI/ARBs, beta-blockers, and lipid-lowering medications.
- The average follow-up was 20 months. The primary end point was death from any cause.

Results

- The incidence of death from any cause was 19.8% in the control group and 14.2% in the treatment group (hazard ratio of 0.69 [95% CI 0.51–0.93; P = 0.016]), indicating a 31% reduction in the risk of death in patients who received an implantable defibrillator.
- The incidence of new or worsened heart failure was slightly higher in the treatment group (19.9%) compared to the control group (14.9%).
- The results were consistent among subgroups of age, sex, ejection fraction, NYHA (New York Heart Association) class, and QRS interval.
- Severe complications related to defibrillator implantation were infrequent.

Importance

Previous studies (MADIT-I [1] and MUSTT [2]) showed that patients with coronary artery disease, reduced left ventricular function, and inducible ventricular arrhythmias on EP studies had survival benefits from defibrillator implantation. These studies required patients to undergo invasive EP studies to determine the risk of arrhythmia prior to the start of the study. However, the prognostic value of EP studies in identifying the patients with advanced heart failure who were at risk of developing significant ventricular arrhythmias was unclear [2]. This study, MADIT-II, showed that in patients with prior history of MI and an EF of 30% or less, implantation of a defibrillator provided a significant mortality benefit without the need to undergo invasive EP study for risk stratification.

In this study, the incidence of new or worsened heart failure was slightly higher in the defibrillator group, likely due to defibrillator shocks leading to myocardial injury and backup ventricular pacing resulting in impaired ventricular function.

Participants with non-ischemic cardiomyopathy were not included in this study, even though the risk of life-threatening ventricular arrhythmia is high in this group [3]. This study did not compare the efficacy of defibrillator and anti-arrhythmic medications in the prevention of ventricular arrhythmias.

Updates

- The DEFINITE trial (2004) showed a statistically significant reduction in sudden death from arrhythmias and a non-significant reduction in death from all cause in patients with non-ischemic cardiomyopathy who underwent implantable cardioverter defibrillator (ICD) implantation compared to conventional medical therapy alone [3].
- The DINAMIT trial (2004) showed that in patients with EF <35% following an acute MI (6–40 days), ICD implantation decreased arrhythmia-related death but did not decrease all-cause mortality when compared to patients on medical therapy alone [4].
- The SCD-Heft study (2006) included patients with ischemic and non-ischemic cardiomyopathy and LVEF < 35%. It compared survival rates in participants receiving either placebo, amiodarone, or an ICD in addition to conventional medical therapy. Results showed that amiodarone had no effect on survival, but the use of an ICD reduced overall mortality by 23% [5].
- The MADIT-CRT trial (2009) showed that in patients with EF < 30%, QRS > 130 s, and NYHA I–III symptoms, ICD implantation with cardiac resynchronization therapy led to improved survival rates compared to ICD implantation alone [6].

Bottom Line

- The use of an implantable defibrillator improves survival rates in patients with a history of myocardial infarction and a left ventricular ejection fraction of <30%.

References

1. Moss AJ, Hall WJ, et al. Improved survival with an implanted defibrillator in patients with coronary disease at high risk for ventricular arrhythmia. N Engl J Med. 1996;335(26):1933–40.
2. Buxton AE, Lee KL, et al. A randomized study of the prevention of sudden death in patients with coronary artery disease. N Engl J Med. 1999;341(25):1882–90.
3. Kadish A, Dyer A, et al. Prophylactic defibrillator implantation in patients with nonischemic dilated cardiomyopathy. N Engl J Med. 2004;350(21):2151–8.

4. Hohnloser SH, Kuck KH, et al. Prophylactic use of an implantable cardioverter-defibrillator after acute myocardial infarction. N Engl J Med. 2004;351(24):2481–8.
5. Bardy GH, Lee KL, et al. Amiodarone or an implantable cardioverter-defibrillator for congestive heart failure. N Engl J Med. 2005;352(3):225–37.
6. Moss AJ, Hall WJ, et al. Cardiac-resynchronization therapy for the prevention of heart-failure events. N Engl J Med. 2009;361(14):1329–38.

Chapter 9
Medical Versus Interventional Management of Stable CAD (COURAGE)-2007

Anne Sprogell

Background

In the few decades leading up to the publishing of this paper, percutaneous coronary intervention (PCI) had become more common as first line intervention for patients with stable coronary artery disease (CAD) even though guidelines still recommended optimal medical therapy (intensive medical therapy, a reduction of risk factors, and lifestyle intervention) as the first line intervention. In 2004, there were more than 1 million procedures to place stents and it was estimated that 85% of all PCI procedures were elective in patients with stable CAD. PCI was known to reduce rates of death or myocardial infarction in patients with acute coronary syndrome, but those benefits had not been shown in patients with stable with CAD.

Objective

The goal of this study, Clinical Outcomes Utilizing Revascularization and Aggressive Drug Evaluation (COURAGE), was to investigate if PCI combined with optimal medical therapy reduced the risk of death and myocardial infarction in patients with stable CAD.

Boden, W. E., Boden, Hochman, J. S., Steg, P. G., Rothe, C., Guan, … Division of Cardiology. (2007, April 12). Optimal Medical Therapy with or without PCI for Stable Coronary Disease: NEJM. Retrieved from https://www.nejm.org/doi/full/10.1056/NEJMoa070829

A. Sprogell (✉)
Jefferson Health, Abington, PA, USA

J. Russell, N. S. Skolnik (eds.), *Top Articles in Primary Care*,
https://doi.org/10.1007/978-3-031-25620-2_9

Design and Methods

- Patients were randomized to either medical management or PCI with medical management.
- Study populations: patients with stable coronary artery disease and patients whose initial Canadian Cardiovascular Society (CCS) Class IV angina stabilized after medical treatment.
- Inclusion criteria: stenosis of 70% or greater in at least one proximal epicardial coronary artery and evidence of ischemia or stenosis of 80% or more and classic angina.
- Exclusion criteria: persistent CCS class IV angina (i.e., angina evoked from minimal activity or at rest), a markedly positive stress test (substantial ST-segment depression or hypotensive response during stage 1 of the Bruce protocol), refractory heart failure or cardiogenic shock, EF < 30%, revascularization in the previous 6 months, and coronary anatomy not suitable for PCI.
- Medical management included aspirin, clopidogrel, metoprolol, amlodipine, isosorbide mononitrate, lisinopril, or losartan; aggressive therapy to lower LDL (with statin or ezetimibe with target LDL 60–85 mg/dl); raising HDL and lowering triglycerides with niacin, fibrates, and exercise.
- Of note, drug-eluting stents were not approved for clinical use until the final 6 months of the study, so few patients had these placed.

Results

- There was no significant difference in primary outcome (death or MI) between those who received optimal medical therapy and those who received optimal medial therapy in addition to PCI.
- The mortality curves between the groups showed no significant difference during the 4.6 year follow-up.
- While the PCI group did show significant decrease in angina at year 1 and 3 of follow-up, there was no significant difference in decrease in angina at year 5.

Update

A recent meta-analysis of all trial comparing revascularization vs optimal medical management concluded, "In patients with stable ischemic heart disease, routine revascularization was not associated with improved survival but was associated with a lower risk of nonprocedural MI and unstable angina with greater freedom from angina at the expense of higher rates of procedural MI" [1].

Importance

A study in 2014 looked at PCI use in stable angina in New Jersey, Maryland, and Florida after the publication of COURAGE trial and found a 17% decrease in the use of PCI. They noted that on average, managing a patient with stable angina with PCI adds $9000 to the cost of treatment of stable angina [2].

Bottom Line

This study demonstrated that there is no significant difference in death or MI rates between optimal medical therapy and optimal medical therapy plus PCI in the treatment of stable coronary artery disease.

References

1. Bangalore S, Maron DJ, Stone GW, Hochman JS. Routine revascularization versus initial medical therapy for stable ischemic heart disease - a systematic review and meta-analysis of randomized trials. Circulation. 2020;142(9):841–57.
2. Howard DH, Shen Y-C. Trends in PCI volume after negative results from the COURAGE trial. Health Serv Res. 2013;49(1):153–70. https://doi.org/10.1111/1475-6773.12082.

Chapter 10
Dabigatran Versus Warfarin in Atrial Fibrillation (RE-LY)-2009

Jeffrey Matthews

Background

Prior to the introduction of direct oral anticoagulants (DOACs), warfarin was the standard oral treatment for anticoagulation for stroke reduction in atrial fibrillation (AFIB). Warfarin presents challenges with practical application requiring frequent monitoring to be kept within a narrow therapeutic range to balance safety and efficacy. A previous study of the DOAC Ximelagatran demonstrated significant hepatotoxicity leaving doubt about DOACs as potential alternatives to Warfarin. The RE-LY trial was the first study to show safety as well as efficacy of DOACs, ushering in a new era of oral anticoagulation.

Objective

The objective of this study was to demonstrate that Dabigatran, a direct thrombin (factor X) inhibitor, was non-inferior to warfarin for anticoagulation in the management of AFIB.

Connolly, S. J., M.D., Ezekowitz, Michael D, MB, ChB., D. Phil, Yusuf, Salim, F.R.C.P.C., D. Phil, Eikelboom, J., M.D., Oldgren, Jonas, M.D., PhD, Parekh, A., M.D., … Wallentin, Lars, M.D., PhD. (2009). Dabigatran versus warfarin in patients with atrial fibrillation. The New England Journal of Medicine, 361(12), 1139–51.
https://www.nejm.org/doi/pdf/10.1056/NEJMoa0905561?articleTools=true.

J. Matthews (✉)
Jefferson Health, Abington, PA, USA

J. Russell, N. S. Skolnik (eds.), *Top Articles in Primary Care*,
https://doi.org/10.1007/978-3-031-25620-2_10

Design and Methods

- 18,113 patients in 951 centers in 44 countries were recruited to receive either Warfarin (non-blinded) or blinded Dabigatran at 110 mg twice per day (BID) or 150 mg of Dabigatran BID.
- Patients were selected based on having a screening positive for AFIB, or if they had AFIB diagnosed within 6 months and had a previous stroke or TIA, LVEF <40%, NYHA II or higher heart failure symptoms within 6 months of screening and an age of 75 or older, or were 65–74 years of age with cardiac risk factors such as diabetes, hypertension, or coronary artery disease.
- Subjects were then followed for 2 years tracking two primary outcomes: stroke and systemic embolism. Major bleeding events were also measured.

Results

- Primary outcome stroke and systemic embolism
  - 150 mg Dabigatran was superior to warfarin for reduction in stroke or systemic embolism with a relative risk (RR) 0.66 ($p < 0.001$). One hundred and ten milligram Dabigatran was non-inferior but not superior to Warfarin with a RR of 0.91 but did not reach significance with a p value of 0.34.
  - Rates of hemorrhagic stroke were significantly lower with both Dabigatran doses with a RR of 0.31 for 110 mg and 0.26 for 150 mg.
- Secondary outcomes mortality and myocardial infarction:
  - Mortality did not differ statistically though the 150 mg of Dabigatran group had a RR of 0.88 with a p value of 0.051, very close to being statistically significant.
  - In the 150 mg Dabigatran group, death from vascular causes was reduced vs. Warfarin with a RR of 0.85 and a p value of 0.04.
  - There was a statistically significant increase in myocardial infarctions in the 150 mg Dabigatran group compared to Warfarin with a RR of 1.38 and a p value of 0.048.
- Bleeding
  - There was a statistically significant reduction in major bleeding events in the 110 mg dabigatran group with a RR of 0.80 and a p value of 0.003. The RR of the 150 mg dose was 0.93 but the p of 0.31 did not reach statistical significance. Further, both groups compared to Warfarin showed reduction in life threatening bleeding, specifically with 110 mg group with a RR of 0.68 and a p value of <0.001 and in the 150 mg group a RR of 0.81 with a p value of 0.04.

- Both Dabigatran groups had a statistically significant reduction in hemorrhagic stroke compared to warfarin. In the 110 mg Dabigatran group they had a RR of 0.38 and in the 150 mg group a RR of 0.26 both had p values <0.001.
- There was a statistically higher risk of GI bleed in both Dabigatran groups compared with warfarin. In the 110 mg Dabigatran group vs. Warfarin the RR was 1.10 and RR was 1.5 in the 150 mg group. The RR was 1.36 between the Dabigatran groups 150 mg vs. 110 mg showing increased GI bleeds with the higher Dabigatran dose.
- Specifically, for intracranial hemorrhage both 110 and 150 mg of Dabigatran showed lower risk versus warfarin with a RR of 0.31 in 110 mg group and 0.40 in the 150 mg group with both p values <0.001. The rate of intracranial bleed was not statistically different between the two dabigatran groups.

- Net Clinical Benefit Outcome
  - Only the 150 mg Dabigatran group showed a net clinical benefit over Warfarin with a RR of stroke, systemic embolism, pulmonary embolism, myocardial infarction, death, and major bleeding of 0.91 with a p value of 0.04. The 110 mg dabigatran had a non statistically significant difference compared to warfarin or compared to the 150 mg Dabigatran group.

Importance

This was the first non-inferiority trial that demonstrated that DOACs are a safe and effective alternative therapy for the treatment of AFIB in those with increased risk for stroke. Compared to warfarin, DOACs do not require monitoring or frequent adjustments. DOACs also have less drug–drug interactions, and a lower risk of fatal intracranial hemorrhage.

Updates

Since the RE-LY trial, two additional trials have shown that compared to Warfarin, the DOACs, specifically Rivaroxaban and Apixaban, (ARISTOTLE trial (Apixaban) and the ROCKET AF trial (Rivaroxaban)), are comparable or better at preventing stroke and systemic embolism with lower or comparable rates of major bleeding events [1]. Reduction in hemorrhagic stroke and all-cause mortality was also seen (a reduction in overall mortality was not found in the RE-LY trial). An observational study conducted by the United States Food and Drug Administration found that dabigatran actually had a similar rate of myocardial infarction and continued to show an increased risk of GI bleed [2]. The RE-LY trial had hypothesized that GI bleeding was related to the acid components of the capsule required to allow uptake of the prodrug in the GI system.

Bottom Line

The RE-LY trial demonstrated that Dabigatran, a direct factor X inhibitor, is non-inferior to Warfarin for anticoagulation in the setting of AFIB with comparable adverse reactions, decreased major bleeding events, and lower incidences of stroke and systemic embolisms.

References

1. Salazar CA, Aguila DD, Cordova EG. Direct thrombin inhibitors versus vitamin K antagonists for preventing cerebral or systemic embolism in people with non-valvular atrial fibrillation. Cochrane Database Syst Rev. 2014;2014(3):CD009893. https://doi.org/10.1002/14651858.cd009893.pub2.
2. FDA. Drug safety communication: FDA study of Medicare patients finds risks lower for stroke. n.d.

Chapter 11
Aspirin and Clopidogrel in Transient Ischemic Attacks (CHANCE)-2013

Ifrah Naeem

Background

Stroke imposes a large burden on global health care resulting in significant mortality and disability [1]. In 2020 the CDC reported stroke as causing one in six cardio vascular deaths in the USA [2]. Ischemic strokes account for a majority of all strokes. A transient ischemic attack (TIA) or a minor stroke poses a high risk of early recurrent stroke event [3]. CHANCE was a large multi-center trial to study incidence of early recurrence of acute ischemic stroke after prompt initiation of dual antiplatelet therapy (DAPT) in patients with TIA and high-risk minor ischemic strokes.

Objective

- To study the effects of early dual antiplatelet therapy with aspirin and clopidogrel vs. aspirin alone on the prevention of early recurrence of stroke after a TIA or minor acute ischemic stroke.

Y. Wang, Y. Wang, X. Zhao, L. Liu, D. Wang, C. Wang, et al. Clopidogrel with aspirin in acute minor stroke or transient ischemic attack. The New England Journal of Medicine. (2013) 369(1), 11–19.
Article PDF: https://www.nejm.org/doi/pdf/10.1056/NEJMoa1215340?articleTools=true.

I. Naeem (✉)
Jefferson Health, Abington, PA, USA
e-mail: Ifrah.Naeem@jefferson.edu

J. Russell, N. S. Skolnik (eds.), *Top Articles in Primary Care*,
https://doi.org/10.1007/978-3-031-25620-2_11

Design and Methods

- CHANCE was a randomized, double-blind, placebo-controlled, multi-center trial conducted in China. Over 5170 patients, between 40 and 90 years of age, presenting within 24 h of onset with acute non-disabling ischemic stroke (defined with NIH stroke scale ≤3) or TIA (ABCD^2 score ≥4) were randomly assigned to either clopidogrel–aspirin or placebo–aspirin arm with a primary endpoint of ischemic or hemorrhagic stroke within 90 days of the follow-up period.
- In the clopidogrel–aspirin group, clopidogrel was initiated as a one-time 300 mg dose followed by daily 75 mg dose along with 75 mg Aspirin for a total of 90 days. Placebo–aspirin arm therapy included a placebo plus 75 mg Aspirin for 90 days.
- Intention to treat analysis was utilized for the study population and difference in new stroke events during the follow-up period was assessed using Kaplan-Meier time-to-event approach.
- Secondary and safety outcomes included a composite of vascular events including stroke, myocardial infarction, vascular death, and moderate to severe bleeding events.

Results

- A statistically significant lower incidence of stroke was recorded in the aspirin–clopidogrel arm in comparison with placebo–aspirin arm (8.2% versus 11.7%) during the follow-up period (hazard ratio, 0.68; $p < 0.001$). A lower rate of fatal or disabling stroke and ischemic stroke was seen in treatment group; however, there was no difference in the incidence of hemorrhagic stroke between the two groups (0.3% each).
- Clopidogrel and aspirin combination did not contribute to increased hemorrhagic events when compared with placebo–aspirin group and no difference in mortality was observed between the study groups.

Importance

CHANCE was one of the pivotal studies supporting early use of short-term DAPT in patients with TIA and minor ischemic stroke as a preventive strategy against recurrent cerebrovascular accidents (CVA). Earlier DAPT trials for stroke prevention showed a statistically insignificant reduction of stroke recurrence (FASTER) and increased bleeding risk (MATCH) [4, 5]. The CHANCE trial successfully examined the efficacy of DAPT for stroke prevention in these patients with a significant reduction in stroke recurrence without increased bleeding risk.

Questions about generalizability have been raised since the CHANCE trial was carried out in a homogeneous population in China. This population has a higher frequency of strokes, uncontrolled risk factors as well as polymorphism in genes regulating the metabolism of clopidogrel [6, 7]. The study reflected a minimal bleeding risk with DAPT due to a short range of therapy, i.e., 90 days, thus an optimal duration required to effectively prevent stroke recurrence with low bleeding risk was not defined by the trial.

Updates

- Owing to the limitations of the CHANCE trial, POINT trial attempted to study DAPT with aspirin and clopidogrel on a large international population. Patients with high-risk TIA and acute minor stroke were enrolled within 12 h of presentation. This study supported the results of the CHANCE trial and showed a reduced composite of stroke, myocardial infarction, and vascular death at 90 days; however, a higher risk of hemorrhage was seen past 90-day treatment [8].
- DAPT using aspirin and ticagrelor was studied in the THALES (2020) trial which supported its use in patients with TIA and acute minor stroke with NIH stroke scale ≤5. Based on the results, FDA recently approved aspirin and ticagrelor for short-term treatment of acute minor ischemic stroke (NIHSS score ≤5) or high-risk TIA [9].
- 2021 American Heart Association/American Stroke Association for secondary stroke prevention guidelines suggest using short-term DAPT for 21 days in patients who present early for acute minor strokes (NIHSS <5) and high-risk TIA (ABCD^2 score >4). A 90-day DAPT regimen is recommended in patients with severe symptomatic intracranial atherosclerosis with stenosis [10].

Bottom Line

- In patients with high-risk TIA or minor ischemic stroke, there is a high risk of recurrence of strokes in the first 24–48 h and then over the subsequent 90 days. In patients who present early, a short-term dual antiplatelet therapy with clopidogrel and aspirin is superior to aspirin monotherapy in reducing the risk of subsequent stroke events.

References

1. Mukherjee D, Patil CG. Epidemiology and the global burden of stroke. World Neurosurg. 2011;76(6, Supplement):S85–90. https://doi.org/10.1016/j.wneu.2011.07.023.

2. Prevention, CfDCa. Underlying cause of death, CDC WONDER Online Database. Centers for Disease Control and Prevention, 1999–2018. Atlanta, GA: Centers for Disease Control and Prevention; 2018. Accessed 12 Mar 2020.
3. Coutts SB, Hill MD, Campos CR, et al. Recurrent events in transient ischemic attack and minor stroke. Stroke. 2008;39(9):2461–6. https://doi.org/10.1161/STROKEAHA.107.513234.
4. Kennedy J, Hill MD, Ryckborst KJ, Eliasziw M, Demchuk AM, Buchan AM. Fast assessment of stroke and transient ischaemic attack to prevent early recurrence (FASTER): a randomised controlled pilot trial. Lancet Neurol. 2007;6(11):961–9. https://doi.org/10.1016/s1474-4422(07)70250-8.
5. Diener HC, Bogousslavsky J, Brass LM, et al. Aspirin and clopidogrel compared with clopidogrel alone after recent ischaemic stroke or transient ischaemic attack in high-risk patients (MATCH): randomised, double-blind, placebo-controlled trial. Lancet. 2004;364(9431):331–7. https://doi.org/10.1016/s0140-6736(04)16721-4.
6. Wang Y, Zhao X, Lin J, et al. Association between CYP2C19 loss-of-function allele status and efficacy of clopidogrel for risk reduction among patients with minor stroke or transient ischemic attack. JAMA. 2016;316(1):70–8. https://doi.org/10.1001/jama.2016.8662.
7. Feldmann E, Daneault N, Kwan E, et al. Chinese-white differences in the distribution of occlusive cerebrovascular disease. Neurology. 1990;40(10):1541–5. https://doi.org/10.1212/wnl.40.10.1540.
8. Johnston SC, Easton JD, Farrant M, et al. Clopidogrel and aspirin in acute ischemic stroke and high-risk TIA. N Engl J Med. 2018;379(3):215–25. https://doi.org/10.1056/NEJMoa1800410.
9. Johnston SC, Amarenco P, Denison H, et al. Ticagrelor and aspirin or aspirin alone in acute ischemic stroke or TIA. N Engl J Med. 2020;383(3):207–17. https://doi.org/10.1056/NEJMoa1916870.
10. Kleindorfer DO, Towfighi A, Chaturvedi S, et al. 2021 Guideline for the prevention of stroke in patients with stroke and transient ischemic attack: a guideline from the American Heart Association/American Stroke Association. Stroke. 2021;52(7):e364–467. https://doi.org/10.1161/STR.0000000000000375.

Chapter 12
Aspirin and Clopidogrel in High-Risk Transient Ischemic Attacks (POINT)-2018

Malik Muhammad Uzair Khan

Background

Roughly 200,000–500,000 cases of transient ischemic attack (TIA) and 795,000 cases of stroke are reported each year in the US [1, 2]. Three-fourths of all stroke cases are first-time events. Stroke is a leading cause of serious long-term disability and mortality worldwide. In patients presenting with high-risk TIAs (ABCD ≥4) or minor ischemic strokes (NIH SS ≤3), there is a high stroke recurrence risk within 48 hours of the index event [3]. The role of early initiation of dual antiplatelet therapy (DAPT) in the prevention of stroke recurrence has been widely studied. POINT trial is a large multicenter trial analyzing the efficacy and side effects of aspirin plus clopidogrel with aspirin monotherapy for secondary prevention of early stroke recurrence in such patients.

Objective

- To compare the efficacy of clopidogrel plus aspirin with aspirin monotherapy, when initiated within 12 h of symptom onset in patients with high-risk TIAs or minor strokes for the prevention of ischemic stroke, myocardial infarction, or

Johnston, S. C., Easton, J. D., Farrant, M., et al. Clopidogrel and Aspirin in Acute Ischemic Stroke and High-Risk TIA. The New England Journal of Medicine, (2018) 379(3), 215–225.
Article PDF: https://www.nejm.org/doi/full/10.1056/nejmoa1800410

M. M. U. Khan (✉)
Jefferson Health, Abington, PA, USA
e-mail: MalikMuhammadUzair.Khan@jefferson.edu

J. Russell, N. S. Skolnik (eds.), *Top Articles in Primary Care*,
https://doi.org/10.1007/978-3-031-25620-2_12

death from ischemic vascular causes at 90 days. It also examines major side effects of these treatment modalities especially major hemorrhage at 90 days.

Designs and Methods

- 4881 participants aged ≥18 years were enrolled in this prospective, intercontinental, multicenter, double-blind, randomized control trial with the primary endpoint as composite of ischemic stroke, myocardial infarction, and ischemic vascular death at 90 days.
- Individuals presenting to the hospital with a high-risk TIA or minor ischemic stroke within 12 h of symptom onset were started on either a combination of clopidogrel (loading dose of 600 mg followed by 75 mg/day of maintenance dose) plus aspirin (dose range of 50–324 mg/day) or an equal dose of aspirin alone. These subjects were followed for 90 days.
- Data was analyzed using an intention-to-treat strategy.
- Patients were also studied for a primary safety outcome of major hemorrhage during the follow-up period.

Results

There was a statistically significant reduction in the primary endpoint of composite vascular death in the clopidogrel-aspirin arm when compared with aspirin monotherapy (incidence of 5.8% vs 6.8%, hazard ratio, 0.75):

- DAPT use was more advantageous in the first 30 days than at 31–90 days in secondary stroke prevention whereas the risk of hemorrhage associated with DAPT use was lower in the first 7 days than at days 8–90.
- At 90-day follow-up, a higher incidence of major bleeding events was reported in the clopidogrel-aspirin arm at 0.9% compared with 0.4% in the aspirin-only arm.
- A significant number of patients were seen to develop major bleeding events leading to the halting of the study in 2017.

Importance

The POINT trial was one of the largest trials studying the efficacy of DAPT in secondary stroke prevention. Before this, the CHANCE trial had reflected similar results, however, had lower generalizability in terms of its population parameters. POINT trial sought to bridge this limitation by enrolling a diverse group of individuals. It also elaborated on the role of DAPT for secondary stroke prevention in the initial 7–30 days vs 31–90 days of the primary event. A pooled data analysis from POINT and CHANCE trials indicated that DAPT was most protective against secondary strokes in the first 21 days after initial presentation with high-risk TIA or acute minor stroke [4]. The POINT trial sought to determine a safe duration of DAPT therapy to avoid bleeding events while optimizing stroke prevention. The American Heart Association/American Stroke Association adopted this as a high-level recommendation in 2019, and it has since then become a standard of care in patients with a qualifying TIA or minor ischemic stroke. The AHA guidelines now say, "In patients presenting with minor noncardioembolic ischemic stroke (NIHSS score ≤3) who did not receive IV alteplase, treatment with dual antiplatelet therapy (aspirin and clopidogrel) started within 24 hours after symptom onset and continued for 21 days is effective in reducing recurrent ischemic stroke for a period of up to 90 days from symptom onset" [5].

Updates

- The THALES trial was completed in 2020 with 11,016 participants, aged ≥40 years. It compared the efficacy of aspirin plus ticagrelor with aspirin plus placebo for the prevention of stroke or death at 30 days after the occurrence of mild-moderate non-cardioembolic stroke (NIHSS ≤ 5) or high-risk TIA (ABCD2 ≥ 6), or symptomatic intracranial or extracranial arterial stenosis. Lower stroke incidence and mortality was seen in the treatment group. FDA approved aspirin and ticagrelor in 2020 as a DAPT for secondary stroke prevention [6].
- A post hoc analysis of the POINT trial determined that DAPT use lowers the risk of ischemic stroke in patients with high-risk TIAs or minor stroke regardless of premorbid antiplatelet use [7].

Bottom Line

There is a lower risk of ischemic stroke, myocardial infarction, or death from an ischemic vascular event in patients with high-risk TIAs or minor strokes who are taking clopidogrel plus aspirin compared to aspirin monotherapy; however, the risk of major hemorrhage increases with extended therapy.

References

1. Roger VL, Go AS, Lloyd-Jones DM, et al. Heart disease and stroke statistics--2012 update: a report from the American Heart Association. Circulation. 2012;125(1):e2–e220. https://doi.org/10.1161/CIR.0b013e31823ac046.
2. Kleindorfer D, Panagos P, Pancioli A, et al. Incidence and short-term prognosis of transient ischemic attack in a population-based study. Stroke. 2005;36(4):720–3. https://doi.org/10.1161/01.STR.0000158917.59233.b7.
3. Erdur H, Scheitz JF, Ebinger M, et al. In-hospital stroke recurrence and stroke after transient ischemic attack. Stroke. 2015;46(4):1031–7. https://doi.org/10.1161/STROKEAHA.114.006886.
4. Pan Y, Elm JJ, Li H, et al. Outcomes associated with Clopidogrel-aspirin use in minor stroke or transient ischemic attack: a pooled analysis of Clopidogrel in high-risk patients with acute non-disabling cerebrovascular events (CHANCE) and platelet-oriented inhibition in new TIA and Minor ischemic stroke (POINT) trials. JAMA Neurol. 2019;76(12):1466–73. https://doi.org/10.1001/jamaneurol.2019.2531.
5. Powers WJ, Rabinstein AA, Ackerson T, et al. Guidelines for the early management of patients with acute ischemic stroke: 2019 update to the 2018 guidelines for the early management of acute ischemic stroke: a guideline for healthcare professionals from the American Heart Association/American Stroke Association. Stroke. 2019;50(12):e344e418. https://doi.org/10.1161/STR.0000000000000211.
6. Johnston SC, Amarenco P, Denison H, et al. Ticagrelor and aspirin or aspirin alone in acute ischemic stroke or TIA. N Engl J Med. 2020;383(3):207–17. https://doi.org/10.1056/NEJMoa1916870.
7. Anadani M, de Havenon A, Henninger N, et al. Antiplatelet use and ischemic stroke risk in minor stroke or transient ischemic attack: a post hoc analysis of the POINT trial. Stroke. 2021;52(12):e773–6. https://doi.org/10.1161/strokeaha.121.035354.

Chapter 13
Dapagliflozin in Low-EF Congestive Heart Failure (DAPA-HF)-2019

Lucy D. Checchio

Background

Previous studies have shown that sodium-glucose co-transporter 2 (SGLT2) inhibitors reduce the risk of hospitalization from heart failure in patients with type 2 diabetes. However, most of the patients in these trials did not have pre-existing heart failure. Therefore, the results primarily suggested that SGLT2 inhibitors can help prevent the development of heart failure in patients with diabetes.

Objective

- To evaluate the efficacy and safety of dapagliflozin in patients with heart failure with reduced ejection fraction (HFrEF), regardless of the presence or absence of diabetes.

McMurray, J., Solomon, S. D., Inzucchi, S. E., et al. (2019). Dapagliflozin in Patients with Heart Failure and Reduced Ejection Fraction. The New England Journal of Medicine, 381(21), 1995–2008.
https://www.nejm.org/doi/full/10.1056/NEJMoa1911303.

L. D. Checchio (✉)
Jefferson Health, Abington, PA, USA
e-mail: Lucy.Checchio@jefferson.edu

J. Russell, N. S. Skolnik (eds.), *Top Articles in Primary Care*,
https://doi.org/10.1007/978-3-031-25620-2_13

Design and Methods

- This was a phase 3, placebo-controlled trial consisting of 4744 participants who had an ejection fraction of 40% or less (average ~31%), New York Heart Association (NYHA) class II, III, or IV symptoms, and a NT-proBNP level of at least 600 pg/mL.
- Participants in both groups were required to have received standard heart failure device and drug therapy (ACE-inhibitor, ARB, or sacubitril-valsartan plus beta-blocker) unless contraindicated. Use of mineralocorticoid receptor antagonists was encouraged.
- Randomization was stratified based on the presence/absence of type 2 diabetes. Forty-five percent of the patients in each group had type 2 diabetes, while fifty-five percent did not.
- The treatment group received dapagliflozin 10 mg daily.
- Assessment included heart failure, volume status, adverse events, Kansas City Cardiomyopathy Questionnaire symptom scores, renal function, and potassium levels. Median duration of follow-up was 18.2 months. Data was evaluated with an intention-to-treat analysis.

Results

- Primary outcomes: worsening heart failure or death from cardiovascular causes occurred in 386 patients (16.3%) in the treatment group compared to 502 patients (21.2%) in the placebo group (hazard ratio, 0.74; $p < 0.001$).
- Cardiovascular death (9.6% dapagliflozin, 11.5% placebo—hazard ratio, 0.82; 95% CI, 0.69–0.98), hospitalization for heart failure (9.7% dapagliflozin, 13.4% placebo), all-cause mortality (11.6% and 13.9%, respectively, hazard ratio, 0.83; 95% CI, 0.71–0.97), worsening of renal function (1.2% dapagliflozin, 1.6% placebo; $p = 0.17$).
- Symptom scores at 8 months were better in the dapagliflozin group.
- Serious renal adverse events, while uncommon, were significantly less frequent in the dapagliflozin group (1% dapagliflozin, 1.9% placebo).
- Effects of dapagliflozin were consistent among most pre-specified subgroups, including patients without diabetes. However, participants in NYHA class III/IV appeared to have less benefit than participants in class II.
- The frequency of adverse events related to volume depletion, renal dysfunction, and hypoglycemia did not differ between groups.

Importance

The DAPA-HF trial differs from previous studies conducted on SGLT2 inhibitors in that all participants had HFrEF and included patients with and without diabetes. This trial also compared participants with diabetes versus those without diabetes.

The DAPA-HF trial demonstrated that the use of dapagliflozin in patients with HRrEF led to a reduced incidence of worsening heart failure and death from cardiovascular causes compared to placebo. Dapagliflozin was as effective in the 55% of patients without type 2 diabetes as in those with diabetes, demonstrating the cardiovascular benefits of SGLT2 inhibitors separate from lowering glucose levels and extending the potential uses of SGLT2 inhibitors to people without diabetes. Use of dapagliflozin did not lead to volume depletion or worsening of renal function, even with the concurrent use of diuretics. All results were substantial, clinically significant, and occurred over a short period of time.

Limitations to this study included the fact that only 5% of participants were black and relatively few were elderly with multiple comorbidities. Only about 1% of participants were in NYHA class IV. The use of sacubitril-valsartan (which has been shown to be more effective than ACE inhibitors/ARBs alone) prior to the study was low.

Updates

- A subsequent study showed that dapagliflozin reduced the risk of ventricular arrhythmias, cardiac arrest, and sudden death when added to conventional therapy in patients with HFrEF [1].
- A 2020 review of the DAPA-HF trial noted that dapagliflozin was similarly effective and safe in patients who were taking sacubitril/valsartan compared to those who were not, suggesting that the use of both agents together could be of benefit in patients with HFrEF [2].
- In the 2020 EMPEROR-Reduced trial, empagliflozin was found to be associated with a lower number of hospitalizations for heart failure and with a slower rate of decline in renal function compared to placebo. This trial included participants with a markedly reduced ejection fraction (mean LVEF 27%) and increased levels of natriuretic peptides, compared to participants in the DAPA-HF trial. This trial extended the benefits of SGLT2 inhibitors to patients with more advanced heart failure [3].
- In the 2022 CHIEF-HF trial, canagliflozin was found to significantly improve symptoms in heart failure, regardless of ejection fraction or diabetes status [4].
- The trial was instrumental in SGLT-2 inhibitors now being recommended in the American Heart Association/American College of Cardiology guidelines on the treatment of heart failure [5].

Bottom Line

- In patients with HFrEF, dapagliflozin was shown to be superior to placebo in lowering the risk of worsening heart failure and death from cardiovascular causes while also resulting in better symptom scores, regardless of diabetes status.

References

1. Curtain JP, Docherty KF, Jhund PS, et al. Effect of dapagliflozin on ventricular arrhythmias, resuscitated cardiac arrest, or sudden death in DAPA-HF. Eur Heart J. 2021;42(36):3727–38.
2. Solomon SD, Jhund PS, Claggett BL, et al. Effect of dapagliflozin in patients with HFrEF treated with sacubitril/valsartan: the DAPA-HF trial. JACC Heart Fail. 2020;8(10):811–8.
3. Packer M, Anker SD, Butler J, et al. Cardiovascular and renal outcomes with empagliflozin in heart failure. N Engl J Med. 2020;383(15):1413–24.
4. Spertus JA, Birmingham MC, Nassif M, et al. The SGLT2 inhibitor canagliflozin in heart failure: the CHIEF-HF remote, patient-centered randomized trial. Nat Med. 2022;28:809. https://doi.org/10.1038/s41591-022-01703-8.
5. Heidenreich P, Bozkurt B, Aguilar D, et al. 2022 AHA/ACC/HFSA guideline for the management of heart failure. J Am Coll Cardiol. 2022;79(17):e263–421. https://doi.org/10.1016/j.jacc.2021.12.012.

Chapter 14
Early Rhythm Control in Atrial Fibrillation (EAST)2020

Rameesha Mehreen

Background

Atrial fibrillation (AF) is the most common arrythmia which is associated with significant morbidity and mortality [1]. Risks associated with atrial fibrillation include transient ischemic attack, strokes, heart failure, and death [2]. Atrial fibrillation is usually treated with rate and rhythm control medications or catheter ablation [3]. The incidence of adverse effects associated with patients suffering from AF is as high as 5% of patients per year [4].

Objective

- To compare the effectiveness of early rhythm control therapy versus usual care in the prevention of adverse cardiovascular events in patients suffering from atrial fibrillation.

Kirchhof, P., Camm, A. J., Goette, A., Brandes, A., Eckardt, L., Elvan, A., Fetsch, T., van Gelder, I. C., Haase, D., Haegeli, L. M., Hamann, F., Heidbüchel, H., Hindricks, G., Kautzner, J., Kuck, K.-H., Mont, L., Ng, G. A., Rekosz, J., Schoen, N., … Breithardt, G. (2020). Early Rhythm-Control Therapy in Patients with Atrial Fibrillation. New England Journal of Medicine, 383(14), 1305–1316.
Hyperlink to PDF: https://doi.org/10.1056/NEJMoa2019422.

R. Mehreen (✉)
Jefferson Health, Abington, PA, USA
e-mail: Rameesha.Mehreen@jefferson.edu

J. Russell, N. S. Skolnik (eds.), *Top Articles in Primary Care*,
https://doi.org/10.1007/978-3-031-25620-2_14

Design and Methods

1. This investigator-driven, multicenter randomized trial included 2789 patients (from 135 sites in 11 European countries). The patient selection criteria included onset of AF (≤12 months prior to randomization) and the risk for stroke evidenced by either:
    (a) *One of the mentioned*: age >75/prior stroke, TIA, ischemic stroke
    (b) *Two of the mentioned*: hypertension, female sex, 65 years, stable heart failure, severe coronary artery disease, left ventricular hypertrophy, diabetes mellitus
2. The patients were randomized to two groups (usual care and rhythm control) for trial interventions. Usual care limited rhythm control to the management of atrial fibrillation-related symptoms. The ratio for randomization was maintained at 1:1 and stratification was done based on sites and grouped by various block lengths. All the participants of the study were given treatment of rate control, anticoagulants, and cardiovascular conditions.
    (a) Usual care (1394 patients): for rate control, patients received primarily beta-blockers and under 5% received digitalis glycosides.
    (b) Early rhythm control (1395 patients): treated with either antiarrhythmic drugs or AF ablation.
3. The treatment outcomes were classified as primary and secondary outcomes.
    Two primary outcomes were evaluated. The first primary outcome was a composite of death from cardiovascular causes, stroke, or hospitalization with worsening of heart failure or acute coronary syndrome; the second primary outcome was the number of nights spent in the hospital per year. The second primary outcome included frequency of hospitalization in terms of the number of nights spent in hospital per year.
    (a) Secondary outcome included each component of first primary outcome as well as the rhythm, AF related symptoms, left ventricular function, assessment of cognitive function, and quality of life.
    (b) Other outcomes included primary-safety-outcome such as death from any cause, stroke, or other complications of rhythm control therapy.

The study focused on event driven trial methods and two statistical software R and Stata were used for the statistical analysis.

Results

1. SR (Sinus Rhythm) occurred more often following early rhythm control treatment compared to the usual care.
2. A first-primary-outcome occurred in 249 patients assigned to early rhythm control (3.9 per 100 person-years) and in 316 patients assigned to usual care (5.0 per 100 person-years) (hazard ratio, 0.79; $p = 0.005$).
3. No significant difference was found for the second primary outcome and primary-safety-outcome between the two groups.
4. The analysis of primary-safety-outcome generated the following results:
   (a) Mortality was similar in two groups; strokes occurred more frequently in the usual care arm, and, while the serious adverse events were more common in the early rhythm control arm, the frequency of these events was low.
5. Secondary outcome evaluation gave no statistical differences between the two groups.

Importance

The AFFIRM study comparing rhythm to rate control showed no significant difference between rate and rhythm control, with a non-significant trend favoring rate control. The EAST-AFNET 4 study enrolled patients early after Afib diagnosis and in contrast to the previously reported studies, the current study made use of AF ablation in combination with antiarrhythmic drugs, demonstrating clinical superiority of rhythm control therapy over usual care without rhythm control.

Updates

- Further comparative analysis on the EAST-AFNET 4 trial has been published recently for early rhythm control therapy in symptomatic vs. asymptomatic patients where no significant difference in the two groups was reported.

Bottom Line

- Less frequent cardiovascular events were associated with early rhythm control therapy than with usual care treatments. The overall safety outcomes associated with both therapies are significantly similar in both treatment groups.

References

1. Prystowsky EN, Padanilam BJ, Fogel RI. Treatment of atrial fibrillation. JAMA. 2015;314(3):278–88. https://doi.org/10.1001/jama.2015.7505.
2. Bordignon S, Chiara Corti M, Bilato C. Atrial fibrillation associated with heart failure, stroke and mortality. J Atr Fibrill. 2012;5(1):467. https://doi.org/10.4022/jafib.467.
3. Frankel G, Kamrul R, Kosar L, Jensen B. Rate versus rhythm control in atrial fibrillation. Can Fam Physician. 2013;59(2):161–8.
4. Willems S, Meyer C, de Bono J, Brandes A, Eckardt L, Elvan A, van Gelder I, Goette A, Gulizia M, Haegeli L, Heidbuchel H, Haeusler KG, Kautzner J, Mont L, Ng GA, Szumowski L, Themistoclakis S, Wegscheider K, Kirchhof P. Cabins, castles, and constant hearts: rhythm control therapy in patients with atrial fibrillation. Eur Heart J. 2019;40(46):3793–3799c. https://doi.org/10.1093/eurheartj/ehz782.

Chapter 15
Empagliflozin in Diastolic Heart Failure (EMPEROR)-2021

Hamza Zahid Ullah Muhammadzai

Background

Heart failure is the inability for the heart to meet the demands of adequate perfusion to the body. Heart failure with preserved ejection fraction (HFpEF) is a subgroup of patients with heart failure who have normal left ventricular ejection fraction (LVEF) with predominantly abnormal diastolic dysfunction, among other pathophysiologic abnormalities [1]. Multiple trials in patients with HFpEF have failed to reach their primary endpoints. The EMPEROR-PRESERVED trial is the first trial to have reach its primary outcome in patients with HFpEF.

Objective

- To compare the effects of empagliflozin (a sodium-glucose cotransporter -2—SGLT2 inhibitor) as compared to placebo to evaluate the outcomes in patients with HFpEF.

Anker, S. D., Butler, J., Filippatos, G., Ferreira, J. P., Bocchi, E., Böhm, M., ... Packer, M. (2021). Empagliflozin in heart failure with a preserved ejection fraction. New England Journal of Medicine, 385(16), 1451–1461.
Hyperlink: https://www.nejm.org/doi/full/10.1056/NEJMoa2107038.

H. Z. U. Muhammadzai (✉)
Jefferson Health, Abington, PA, USA
e-mail: Hamza.Muhammadzai@jefferson.edu

J. Russell, N. S. Skolnik (eds.), *Top Articles in Primary Care*,
https://doi.org/10.1007/978-3-031-25620-2_15

Design and Methods

- The study included 5988 patients at 622 centers in 23 countries in a randomized, double blinded multicenter trial.
- Patients were assigned randomly in a 1:1 ratio, with one group receiving 10 mg empagliflozin and the other group receiving placebo.
- Primary outcome was a composite of cardiovascular death or hospitalization for heart failure.
- Patients randomized to have equal distribution of patients in both study arms based on sex, age, race, geographic distribution, New York Heart Association (NYHA) functional classification, pro-BNP, LVEF, diabetes status, e-GFR, and other baseline characteristics.
- Primary outcome was evaluated in an intention-to-treat analysis.
- Patients were followed up for a total of 36 months and a median of 26.2 months.

Results

- The study reached statistical significance for the primary outcome with 6.9 events per 100 patient-years in the empagliflozin group vs. 8.7 events per 100 in placebo (HR 0.79–95% CI 0.69–0.90, $p < 0.001$).
- Absolute risk of hospitalization from heart failure in the empagliflozin group vs. placebo group was reduced (8.6% vs. 11.8%: HR 0.71–95% CI 0.60–0.83).
- Mortality benefit was seen in the intervention group but was not statistically significant (7.3% vs. 8.2%: HR 0.91–95% CI 0.76–1.09).
- Numbers needed to treat (NNT) to prevent one primary outcome was 31.
- Benefits were seen whether patients were diabetic or nondiabetic.
- Secondary outcomes of total number of heart failure hospitalizations and rate of eGFR decline also reduced in intervention group and were statistically significant.

Importance

The EMPEROR-Preserved trial is the first trial to show benefit in patients with HFpEF by preventing hospitalizations due to heart failure. Conversely, previous trials studying the benefits of SGLT-2 inhibitors in patient with HFrEF including the DAPA-HF [2] and EMPEROR-Reduced [3] have shown benefits by reducing the risk of worsening heart failure or death from cardiovascular causes with dapagliflozin and reducing hospitalization from heart failure in patients taking empagliflozin respectively.

It is important to note that other trials in patients with HFpEF including CHARM-Preserved in 2003 [4] (candesartan vs. placebo), I-PRESEVE [5] in 2008 (irbesartan vs. placebo), TOPCAT in 2014 [6] (spironolactone vs. placebo), PARAGON-HF in 2019 [7] (sacubitril-valsartan vs. placebo) failed to reach primary outcomes of reduction in cardiovascular morality.

Updates

- In February 2022, based largely on the results of the results of the EMPEROR-PRESERVED trial, the FDA expanded the indication for empagliflozin to include patients with HFpEF.
- PRESERVED-HF [8] (the SGLT2 inhibitor dapagliflozin in heart failure with preserved ejection fraction) compared the effects of dapagliflozin vs. placebo to evaluate improvements in quality of life and symptom improvement in patients with heart failure. This trial met its primary outcome of improvement in the Kansas City Cardiomyopathy Questionnaire Clinical Summary Score (KCCQ-CS) at 12 weeks, including improvement in symptoms and physical limitations. There was also a statistically significant improvement in the distance walked in the 6-min walk test.
- Top line results of the DELIVER trial of dapagliflozin in HFpEF were released in May 2022 showing that dapagliflozin, "met its primary endpoint in the DELIVER phase III trial by significantly lowering the risk of cardiovascular death or worsening heart failure in patients with mildly reduced or preserved ejection fraction (HFpEF)."

Bottom Line

- The use of SGLT-2 inhibitors in patients with HFrEF and HFpEF has proven beneficial in multiple trials including the EMPEROR-Preserved trial irrespective of diabetes status. Hence, their use in the primary treatment of diabetes should be re-evaluated and extended to patients with heart failure.

References

1. Oktay AA, Rich JD, Shah SJ. The emerging epidemic of heart failure with preserved ejection fraction. Curr Heart Fail Rep. 2013;10(4):401–10.
2. McMurray JJ, Solomon SD, Inzucchi SE, Køber L, Kosiborod MN, Martinez FA, et al. Dapagliflozin in patients with heart failure and reduced ejection fraction. N Engl J Med. 2019;381(21):1995–2008.

3. Packer M, Anker SD, Butler J, Filippatos G, Pocock SJ, Carson P, et al. Cardiovascular and renal outcomes with empagliflozin in heart failure. N Engl J Med. 2020;383(15):1413–24.
4. Yusuf S, Pfeffer MA, Swedberg K, Granger CB, Held P, McMurray JJ, Michelson EL, Olofsson B, Ostergren J, CHARM Investigators and Committees. Effects of candesartan in patients with chronic heart failure and preserved left-ventricular ejection fraction: the CHARM-preserved trial. Lancet. 2003;362(9386):777–81. https://doi.org/10.1016/S0140-6736(03)14285-7.
5. Massie BM, Carson PE, McMurray JJ, Komajda M, McKelvie R, Zile MR, et al. Irbesartan in patients with heart failure and preserved ejection fraction. N Engl J Med. 2008;359(23):2456–67.
6. Pitt B, Pfeffer MA, Assmann SF, Boineau R, Anand IS, Claggett B, et al. Spironolactone for heart failure with preserved ejection fraction. N Engl J Med. 2014;370:1383–92.
7. Solomon SD, McMurray JJ, Anand IS, Ge J, Lam CS, Maggioni AP, et al. Angiotensin–neprilysin inhibition in heart failure with preserved ejection fraction. N Engl J Med. 2019;381(17):1609–20.
8. Nassif ME, Windsor SL, Borlaug BA, Kitzman DW, Shah SJ, Tang F, et al. The SGLT2 inhibitor dapagliflozin in heart failure with preserved ejection fraction: a multicenter randomized trial. Nat Med. 2021;27(11):1954–60.

Part III
Diabetes

Neil Skolnik

Chapter 16
Discovery of Insulin-1922

Alex Scott Fierstein

Background

In 1889 von Mering and Minkowski demonstrated a link between the pancreas and diabetes by removing whole pancreases from dogs that subsequently developed severe and fatal diabetes. Over the decades following, investigators produced various extracts derived from animal pancreases seeking to isolate the agent presumed to oppose the harmful effects of diabetes. At the time it was known the acinous enzyme-secreting portion of the pancreas was destructive to the islet tissue responsible for carbohydrate metabolism when extracts were derived from whole pancreas. Ibrahim is considered the first person to observe that the pancreases of fetal calves under 5 months gestation were almost entirely comprised of islet tissue and devoid of the proteolytic tissue. Banting and Best took advantage of such potent and readily available tissue by administering daily injections of the fetal extracts to a diabetic dog (Marjorie), extending its life by 72 days, whereas untreated diabetic dogs did not live longer than 14 days. Collip then went on to produce a potent, sterile extract suitable for human subjects.

Banting, F. G., Best, C. H., Collip, J. B., Campbell, W. R., & Fletcher, A. A. (1922). Pancreatic Extracts in the Treatment of Diabetes Mellitus. Canadian Medical Association Journal, 12(3), 141–146.
Hyperlink to PDF: https://www.ncbi.nlm.nih.gov/pmc/articles/PMC1524425/.

A. S. Fierstein (✉)
Jefferson Health, Abington, PA, USA
e-mail: alex.fierstein@jefferson.edu

J. Russell, N. S. Skolnik (eds.), *Top Articles in Primary Care*,
https://doi.org/10.1007/978-3-031-25620-2_16

Objective

To study the effects of extracts from the pancreases of fetal calves and adult cows on humans with diabetes.

Design and Methods

- The researchers performed an uncontrolled trial studying the effects of pancreatic extracts on seven subjects admitted to the medical ward of Toronto General Hospital, each with varying severities of diabetes mellitus.
- Each subject was placed on a consistent diet personalized to his/her severity of illness for 1 week, during which the following parameters were assessed:
  - Routine history and physical examination
  - 24-h urine glucose (g)
  - Blood sugar (mg/cm^3)
  - Quantitative urine acetone (mg/L)
  - Qualitative urine acetone
  - Respiratory quotient
- Following 1 week on diet alone, various, unspecified concentrations of pancreatic extracts were administered at various, unspecified intervals while continuing to observe the above listed parameters.
- The study presents a case report of one subject in greater detail: a 14-year-old male with a 2-year history of diabetes mellitus admitted to Toronto General on December 2nd, 1921, for clinical signs and evidence of diabetic ketoacidosis.
- The subject's past medical history included otorrhea during infancy and varicella at age 10; his immediate relatives were in good health and there was no family history of diabetes.
- After initial observation on diet alone, the subject received 15 cm^3 of an unconcentrated form of extract on the evening of January 11, 1922.
- The effects were observed for 11 days without further treatment.
- Beginning January 23rd, the subject received twice daily injections of more concentrated extract on 11 out of the next 13 days.
- Following the daily treatment period the subject was observed for 11 days without any treatment.
- On February 16th the subject again received concentrated extract for three of the next 5 days.

Results

- Measured 2 days pre-treatment and 1 day post-treatment, the subject's 24-h urine glucose decreased from 126.7 to 84 g; blood sugar from 6.2 to 4.9 mg/cm^3; urine acetone from 540 to 69 mg/L.
- On the days following initial treatment, all parameters returned to pre-treatment levels.
- During the 13-day treatment period, urine glucose varied between 7.5 and 45.1 g and ketonuria disappeared.
- Measured on a less frequent basis, blood sugar dropped from 5.2 mg/cm^3 on day 1 of daily treatment to 1.2–3.0 mg/cm^3 on day 2.
- During this period, the subject exhibited notably more energy, strength, and vigor than prior to treatment.
- During the next 11-day period without treatment, all measured parameters again began returning to pre-treatment levels.
- The final 5-day treatment period at the end of subject's case again demonstrated decreased urinary glucose, blood sugar, and ketonuria.
- All six other subjects were noted to improve clinically as well.

Importance

Over 100 years since the first successful human application of a purified pancreatic extract come to be known as the hormone insulin, it may be impossible to overstate the potent and everlasting contribution this 1922 study provided modern medicine. Prior to the discovery of insulin, type I patients lived, on average, 10 months after their diabetes diagnosis. Accounting for both type 1 and type 2 diabetes, one in ten individuals aged 20–79 years are living with diabetes worldwide, a figure that currently represents 537 million adults and is expected to rise to 643 million by 2030 and to 783 million by 2045 [1]. In 2021 diabetes accounted for 6.7 million deaths worldwide [1]. Furthermore, 541 million adults currently have impaired glucose tolerance, placing them at high risk for developing type 2 diabetes [1]. Though several classes of non-insulin antidiabetic medications are widely used in the treatment of type 2 diabetes, the number of type 2 diabetics requiring insulin are projected to increase by over 20% between 2018 and 2030 [2]. Today insulin remains the only definitive treatment for type 1 diabetes and is a critical treatment for a significant proportion of type 2 diabetes. It is for these reasons insulin has been on the World Health Organization's List of Essential Medications since the list was first published in 1977.

Bottom Line

This study first proved that insulin derived from bovine pancreas can safely be administered in human diabetics to reverse diabetic ketoacidosis.

References

1. International Diabetes Federation. IDF diabetes atlas. 10th ed. Brussels: International Diabetes Federation; 2021.
2. Basu S, Yudkin JS, Kehlenbrink S, Davies J, Lipska KJ, Sussman JB, Beran D. Estimation of global insulin use for type 2 diabetes mellitus, 2018-2030. Amsterdam: Health Action International; 2018. https://accisstoolkit.haiweb.org/wp-content/uploads/2020/10/Estimate-of-Insulin-Use-in-Type-2-Diabetes1.pdf. Accessed 14 Apr 2022.

Chapter 17
Diabetes Control and Outcomes (DCCT)-1993

Bhasha Mukhopadhyay

Background

Prior to this study it was well known that IDDM led to both microvascular and macrovascular complications over time. It was believed that sustained hyperglycemia was a critical factor in the pathogenesis of those complications, but there was not direct evidence that long-term control of blood sugars decreased the incidence of these complications. This study was designed to examine whether intensive treatment of insulin-dependent diabetes mellitus (IDDM) with a goal of maintaining blood glucose close to normal range could decrease the frequency and severity of complications [1].

Objective

- To determine whether intensive treatment of IDDM will slow the onset and progression of complications of diabetes such as retinopathy, nephropathy, and neuropathy.

The Diabetes Control and Complications Trial Research Group. (1993). The Effect of Intensive Treatment of Diabetes on the Development and Progression of Long-Term Complications in Insulin-Dependent Diabetes Mellitus. New England Journal of Medicine, 329(14), 977–986. https://doi.org/10.1056/nejm199309303291401.
Hyperlink to PDF: https://www.nejm.org/doi/pdf/10.1056/NEJM199309303291401?articleTools=true.

B. Mukhopadhyay (✉)
Jefferson Health Abington, Abington, PA, USA
e-mail: Bhasha.Mukhopadhyay@jefferson.edu

J. Russell, N. S. Skolnik (eds.), *Top Articles in Primary Care*,
https://doi.org/10.1007/978-3-031-25620-2_17

Design and Methods

- Neither patients nor investigators knew outcome data unless the predetermined criteria were met; at that point, physician and patient were told the specific condition and arranged for appropriate management.
- 1441 patients total recruited at 29 centers, between 1983 and 1989
- Eligibility criteria:
  - Insulin dependence (deficient C-peptide secretion)
  - Age 13–39 years
  - Absence of hypertension, hypercholesterolemia, and severe diabetic complications or medical conditions
  - Primary cohort required to have IDDM for 1–5 years, no retinopathy, urinary albumin excretion <40 mg/24 h
  - Secondary intervention cohort required to have IDDM for 1–15 years, very mild to moderate non-proliferative retinopathy, urinary albumin excretion <200 mg/24 h
- Conventional therapy group:
  - Included 1–2 daily injections of insulin (mixed intermediate and rapid-acting), daily self-monitoring of urine or blood glucose, and dietary and exercise counseling
  - Goals were absence of symptoms due to glycosuria or hyperglycemia, absence of ketonuria, maintenance of normal growth/development/body weight, freedom from severe or frequent hypoglycemia
  - Examined every 3 months
- Intensive therapy group:
  - Administration of insulin 3 or more times daily by injection or external pump, dosage adjusted according to blood glucose, diet, and exercise
  - Goals were preprandial blood glucose 70–120 mg/dL, postprandial <180 mg/dL, weekly 3 AM measurement >65 mg/dL, HbA1C measured monthly within normal range (<6.05%)
  - Visited study center each month and contacted by telephone even more frequently for regimen review and adjustments if necessary

Results

- The cohort was followed for a mean of 6.5 years.
- The mean value for all glucose profiles in the intensive therapy group was 155 mg/dL vs. 231 mg/dL in the conventional therapy group. The average A1c during the first 3 years of the study was just under 7% in the intensive therapy group vs. approximately 9% in the conventional therapy group. During the rest

of the study the A1c in the intensive therapy group was approximately in the intensive therapy group vs. 9% in the conventional therapy group.

- Intensive therapy shown to delay onset and slow progression of retinopathy, nephropathy, and neuropathy complications, by more than 35–70%.
- Intensive therapy reduced risk of albuminuria and microalbuminuria.
- Intensive therapy reduced the development of neuropathy.
- The relatively young age of the group made the detection of a difference in macrovascular outcomes unlikely. When cardiovascular and peripheral vascular events were combined, intensive therapy reduced the incidence of macrovascular disease by 41%, which did not reach statistical significance.
- Intensive therapy group had risk of severe hypoglycemia that was three times higher than the standard therapy group; though few patients required hospitalization due to this and they all had no changes in cognitive function
- The authors concluded that the risk of severe hypoglycemia with intensive therapy was greatly outweighed by reduction in microvascular and neurologic complications
- Due to risk of severe hypoglycemia, the authors pointed out the "risk–benefit ratio with intensive therapy may be less favorable" in children <13 years of age. Patients with advanced complications such as end-stage renal/cardiovascular/cerebrovascular disease, and in patients with advanced complications. Also, it was noted that patients with proliferative or severe non-proliferative retinopathy may be at higher risk of progression of their retinopathy in an accelerated fashion shortly after starting intensive therapy

Importance

The DCCT was the first study to show that intensive glucose lowering therapy in patients with insulin-dependent diabetes mellitus slowed the onset and progression of diabetic complications.

Bottom Line

- Intensive therapy (as listed above) slows the onset and progression of complications of diabetes mellitus such as retinopathy, nephropathy, and neuropathy in patients with insulin-dependent diabetes mellitus.

Reference

1. The Diabetes Control and Complications Trial Research Group. The effect of intensive treatment of diabetes on the development and progression of long-term complications in insulin-dependent diabetes mellitus. N Engl J Med. 1993;329(14):977–86. https://doi.org/10.1056/nejm199309303291401.

Chapter 18
Lifestyle and Diabetes Prevention (DPP)-2002

Angela Kalinowski

Background

Type 2 diabetes affects approximately 14% of adults in the USA. There are many known risk factors for developing diabetes, some of which are reversible, including being overweight and living a sedentary lifestyle. Treatment of diabetes can prevent some of its lasting consequences; however, preventing the progression to diabetes would be preferable. At the time of a diagnosis of diabetes, complications are often already present [1]. Diabetes affected an estimated 171 million people worldwide in 2000, and this number is projected to rise to 366 million by 2030, due in part to increases in age, obesity, and urbanization of the population [2].

Objective

The objective of this study was to determine if modifying the risk factors for diabetes with a lifestyle intervention program or the administration of metformin could prevent or delay the development of diabetes in adults who were at high risk for the

---

Knowler, W. C., Barrett-Connor, E., Fowler, S. E., Hamman, R. F., Lachin, J. M., Walker, E. A., … Diabetes Prevention Program Research Group (2002). Reduction in the incidence of type 2 diabetes with lifestyle intervention or metformin. The New England journal of medicine, 346(6), 393–403. doi:10.1056/NEJMoa012512. https://www.ncbi.nlm.nih.gov/pmc/articles/PMC1370926/.

A. Kalinowski (✉)
Jefferson Health, Abington, PA, USA

J. Russell, N. S. Skolnik (eds.), *Top Articles in Primary Care*,
https://doi.org/10.1007/978-3-031-25620-2_18

development of type 2 diabetes. The study aimed to determine if these two methods (lifestyle intervention vs. metformin) differed in effectiveness and if the effectiveness varied based on age, sex, race, or ethnic group.

Design and Methods

- 3234 persons without a diagnosis of diabetes but with elevated fasting and post load plasma glucose concentrations were randomly assigned to placebo plus standard lifestyle recommendations, metformin plus standard lifestyle recommendations, or an intensive lifestyle modification program arm of the trial.
- Eligibility criteria included age >25 years, BMI of 24 or greater, a fasting plasma glucose of 95–125 mg/dL, and plasma glucose of 140–199 mg/dL 2 h after a 75 g oral glucose load.
- Metformin was administered at a dose of 850 mg once daily and increased to twice daily at 1 month.
- Standard lifestyle recommendations were provided via written information and an annual 30 min information session. Participants were told to follow the Food Guide Pyramid and the equivalent of a National Cholesterol Education Step 1 diet to reduce their weight and to increase their physical activity.
- The lifestyle modification program included goals of at least 7% weight loss through healthy low-calorie, low-fat diet and 150 min of moderate intensity physical activity per week. Participants were given a 16 lesson curriculum covering diet, exercise, and behavior modification that was taught on an individualized one-to-one basis.
- Participants were screened for the development of diabetes on an annual basis based on oral glucose tolerance test or semi-annual fasting plasma glucose value. Diabetes was diagnosed based on fasting plasma glucose value of 126 mg/dL or higher or plasma glucose level of 200 mg/dL or higher 2 h after a 75 g oral glucose load. The diagnosis was confirmed by a second test with the same criteria within 6 weeks.
- Participants self-reported levels of physical activity annually via questionnaire. Daily calorie intake, including calories from fats, carbs, protein, other nutrients, was assessed at baseline and at 1 year with a questionnaire.

Results

- The participants in the study were followed for an average of 2.8 years.
- 50% of the participants in the lifestyle intervention group had attained the goal of 7% weight loss by the end of the 24 week curriculum, and 38% had a weight loss of at least 7% at their most recent visit. Seventy-four percent of participants in this arm of the trial met the 150 min goal of physical activity per week at 24 weeks and 58% at their most recent visit.

- 97% of the participants taking placebo and 84% of those assigned metformin were given the full dose of one tablet twice a day, the remainder were given one tablet daily to limit side effects.
- The average weight loss was 0.1 kg in the placebo group, 2.1 kg in the metformin group, and 5.6 kg in the lifestyle intervention group.
- **The incidence of diabetes was 58% lower in the lifestyle intervention group and 31% lower in the metformin group than in the placebo group.**
- The incidence of diabetes was 39% lower in the lifestyle intervention group than in the metformin group.
- The effects of the treatment did not significantly differ according to either sex, race, or ethnic group.

Importance

This study supported the theory that type 2 diabetes can be prevented in those people at high risk to develop the disease. The study proved that this reduction in incidence can be achieved through intensive diet and exercise alone and did not require medication intervention. Metformin was found to be effective in preventing progression to diabetes, however, less so than lifestyle changes.

Updates

- 88% of the participants enrolled in the above Diabetes Prevention Program (DPP) trial enrolled for additional follow-up of a mean of 5.7 years, termed the Diabetes Prevention Program Outcomes Study (DPPOS). Incidence rates were stable in the lifestyle group, but fell in the placebo and metformin groups during the DPPOS. During the combined DPP, bridge, and DPPOS periods, the incidence rate of the lifestyle group was reduced by 34% and metformin by 18% compared with placebo. The cumulative incidence of diabetes remained the lowest in the lifestyle intervention group. This study proved prevention or delay of diabetes with lifestyle intervention or metformin can persist for at least 10 years [2].
- A 15 year follow-up study was completed to assess whether the interventions studied in the DPP reduced diabetes associated microvascular complication. During a mean follow-up of 15 years, diabetes incidence was reduced by 27% in the lifestyle intervention group and by 18% in the metformin group compared with the placebo group. The prevalence at the end of the study of the aggregate microvascular outcome (nephropathy, retinopathy, and neuropathy) was not significantly different between the treatment groups in the total cohort [3].
- Results of the DPPT have been used to develop programs certified by the CDC that have been implemented throughout the United States [4].

Bottom Line

In adults who are at high risk for development of type 2 diabetes, intensive lifestyle interventions are effective at decreasing progression to diabetes and were shown to be more effective in reducing the incidence of progression to diabetes than treatment with metformin.

References

1. Knowler WC, Barrett-Connor E, Fowler SE, Hamman RF, Lachin JM, Walker EA, et al. Reduction in the incidence of type 2 diabetes with lifestyle intervention or metformin. N Engl J Med. 2002;346(6):393–403. https://doi.org/10.1056/NEJMoa012512.
2. Diabetes Prevention Program Research Group, Knowler WC, Fowler SE, Hamman RF, Christophi CA, Hoffman HJ, et al. 10-year follow-up of diabetes incidence and weight loss in the Diabetes Prevention Program Outcomes Study. Lancet. 2009;374(9702):1677–86. https://doi.org/10.1016/S0140-6736(09)61457-4.
3. Diabetes Prevention Program Research Group. Long-term effects of lifestyle intervention or metformin on diabetes development and microvascular complications over 15-year follow-up: the Diabetes Prevention Program Outcomes Study. Lancet Diabetes Endocrinol. 2015;3(11):866–75. https://doi.org/10.1016/S2213-8587(15)00291-0.
4. The National Diabetes Prevention Program. https://www.cdc.gov/diabetes/prevention/index.html.

Chapter 19
Tight Control of Diabetes in Adult Patients (ACCORD)-2008

Juliana Carvajal and Gregory Palko

Background

Diabetes mellitus leads to both microvascular and macrovascular complications. Microvascular complications include nephropathy, retinopathy, and neuropathy. Macrovascular complications include coronary artery disease, stroke, and peripheral vascular disease. Epidemiologic studies had shown that the incidence of these complications is related to the degree of hyperglycemia. By the early 2000s previous randomized prospective studies had shown that decreasing the degree of hyperglycemia could decrease the incidence of microvascular disease. Two data gaps remained. There remained a paucity of data on the effect of lowering blood sugar on macrovascular outcomes. It was also unclear whether very tight control of blood sugars yielded a benefit beyond that of moderate control of blood sugars [1].

Objective

- The ACCORD trial was designed to determine if a strategy targeting normal glycated hemoglobin levels (below 6.0%) would reduce the rate of cardiovascular events, compared to a strategy targeting glycated hemoglobin levels from 7.0

Gerstein, H.C., Miller, M. E., et al. *Effects of Intensive Glucose Lowering in Type 2 Diabetes, The New England Journal of Medicine 2008;* 358:2545-2559.
Hyperlink to PDF: https://www.nejm.org/doi/full/10.1056/nejmoa0802743.

J. Carvajal (✉) · G. Palko
Jefferson Health, Abington, PA, USA
e-mail: juliana.carvajal@jefferson.edu; Gregory.Palko@jefferson.edu

J. Russell, N. S. Skolnik (eds.), *Top Articles in Primary Care*,
https://doi.org/10.1007/978-3-031-25620-2_19

to 7.9% in middle age and older adults with type two diabetes mellitus who either had underlying vascular disease or multiple risk factors for vascular disease.

Design and Methods

- Participants recruited had type 2 diabetes and were:
  - Between the ages of 40 and 79 and had cardiovascular disease
  - Between the ages of 55 and 79 and had evidence of atherosclerosis or two risk factors for heart disease
- A total of 10,251 participants were randomly assigned to either intensive therapy group or a standard therapy group
  - Intensive therapy aimed to have a glycated hemoglobin level less than 6%
  - Standard therapy aimed to have a glycated hemoglobin of 7–7.9%
- Of those 10,251, 4733 were randomly assigned to an intensive therapy group to lower blood pressure vs. standard therapy to lower blood pressure
  - Intensive therapy to lower blood pressure aimed for a systolic blood pressure less than 120 mmHg
  - Standard therapy to lower blood pressure aimed for a systolic blood pressure less than 140 mmHg
- Of those 10,251 participants, 5518 were placed in a category to maintain low density lipoprotein control and then assigned to either receive fenofibrate or a placebo to study the effect of lowering triglycerides

Results

- The intensive therapy group dropped to a median of glycated hemoglobin of 6.4% and standard therapy decreased to 7.5% in 1 year
- During follow-up there was a non-significant trend favoring the intensive therapy group in the primary outcome of a composite of nonfatal myocardial infarction, nonfatal stroke, or death from cardiovascular causes (hazard ratio, 0.90; $P = 0.16$)
- Compared to the standard therapy group, intensive therapy had a greater rate of hypoglycemia
- The intensive therapy group had a greater rate of death from cardiovascular causes compared to the standard therapy group

- After 3.5 years, death rates were seen to be higher in the intensive therapy group so the study was discontinued due to safety concerns
- Subgroup analysis showed that patients in the intensive therapy group who had not had a cardiovascular event before randomization or whose baseline A1c ≤ 8.0% had fewer fatal or nonfatal cardiovascular events than did patients in the standard therapy group, favoring intensive therapy for this group of patients.

Importance

The ACCORD study raised many questions. It was anticipated that this study would show that intensive therapy to bring blood glucose down to near normal levels would yield a benefit that was greater than standard therapy. The study showed that in the group of patients studied, those with long-standing diabetes many of whom had underlying CV disease with an average A1c of 8.3, intensive therapy increased mortality. The questions were raised by the details. Subgroup analysis showed that intensive therapy yielded a better outcome than standard therapy in patients who did not already have underlying CV disease and who had better A1c (≤8%) on entry to the study. In addition, intensive therapy did decrease the incidence of progression of nephropathy. This study, along with the results of additional studies including ADVANCE and VADT lead to the recommendation to individualize A1c goals [2, 3]. Individualized goals meant that younger patients who have a shorter duration of diabetes with few comorbidities are now recommended to have lower A1c targets, and older patients who have a longer duration of diabetes, particularly underlying CV disease, to have a target A1c that is not as low.

Updates

- The results of additional studies including ADVANCE and VADT as well as long-term follow-up of these studies goes beyond the scope of this review.
- Five-year follow up of the ACCORD study showed results similar to the initial study [4].
- It was found that combination lipid therapy with fenofibrate and simvastatin did not reduce the rate of cardiovascular events or strokes compared to simvastatin alone [6].
- As for hypertension, the intensive therapy group had higher rates of adverse events, hypokalemia, and increased creatinine levels but overall neither group showed a significant reduction in cardiovascular events [1].

Bottom Line

- Glycemic goals need to be individualized. The current American Diabetes Association Standards of Care recommend: "An *A1C goal for many nonpregnant adults of <7%* without significant hypoglycemia. On the basis of provider judgment and patient preference, achievement of lower A1C levels than the goal of 7% may be acceptable and even beneficial if it can be achieved safely without significant hypoglycemia or other adverse effects of treatment. *Less stringent A1C goals* such as <8% may be appropriate for patients with *limited life expectancy*, or where the harms of treatment are greater than the benefits [5]."
- There is no real significant decrease of cardiovascular risk with fenofibrate and simvastatin vs. simvastatin alone when it comes to lipid therapy [6]
- There is no significant evidence that targeting a systolic blood pressure of 140 mmHg versus 120 mmHg reduces major cardiovascular events in type 2 diabetes [7]

References

1. UK Prospective Diabetes Study (UKPDS) Group. Intensive blood-glucose control with sulphonylureas or insulin compared with conventional treatment and risk of complications in patients with type 2 diabetes (UKPDS 33). Lancet. 1998;352:837–53. [Erratum, Lancet 1999;354:602.]
2. The ADVANCE Collaborative Group. Intensive blood glucose control and vascular outcomes in patients with type 2 diabetes. N Engl J Med. 2008;358:2560–72.
3. Duckworth W, Abraira C, Moritz T, et al. Glucose control and vascular complications in veterans with type 2 diabetes. N Engl J Med. 2009;360:129–39.
4. ACCORD Study Group, Gerstein HC, Miller ME, Genuth S, Ismail-Beigi F, Buse JB, Goff DC Jr, Probstfield JL, Cushman WC, Ginsberg HN, Bigger JT, Grimm RH Jr, Byington RP, Rosenberg YD, Friedewald WT. Long-term effects of intensive glucose lowering on cardiovascular outcomes. N Engl J Med. 2011;364(9):818–28. https://doi.org/10.1056/NEJMoa1006524.
5. Dluhy RG, McMahon GT. Intensive glycemic control in the ACCORD and ADVANCE trials. N Engl J Med. 2008;358:2630–3. https://doi.org/10.1056/NEJMoa0804182.
6. ACCORD Study Group, Ginsberg HN, Elam MB, Lovato LC, Crouse JR III, Leiter LA, Linz P, Friedewald WT, Buse JB, Gerstein HC, Probstfield J, Grimm RH, Ismail-Beigi F, Bigger JT, Goff DC Jr, Cushman WC, Simons-Morton DG, Byington RP. Effects of combination lipid therapy in type 2 diabetes mellitus. N Engl J Med. 2010;362(17):1563–74. https://doi.org/10.1056/NEJMoa1001282.
7. ACCORD Study Group, Cushman WC, Evans GW, Byington RP, Goff DC Jr, Grimm RH Jr, Cutler JA, Simons-Morton DG, Basile JN, Corson MA, Probstfield JL, Katz L, Peterson KA, Friedewald WT, Buse JB, Bigger JT, Gerstein HC, Ismail-Beigi F. Effects of intensive blood-pressure control in type 2 diabetes mellitus. N Engl J Med. 2010;362(17):1575–85. https://doi.org/10.1056/NEJMoa1001286.

Chapter 20
Blood Sugar Control in Intensive Care Patients (NICE SUGAR)-2009

Angela Kalinowski

Background

Hyperglycemia is common in acutely ill patients and is associated with increased mortality in some groups of patients. Based largely on a trial which demonstrated that an intensive intravenous insulin regimen to reach a target glycemic range of 80–110 mg/dL reduced mortality by 40% compared with a standard approach targeting blood glucose of 180–215 mg/dL in critically ill patients with recent surgery many professional organizations were recommending tight glucose control [1].

Objective

To test the hypothesis that intensive glucose control reduces mortality at 90 days in critically ill patients.

Intensive versus Conventional Glucose Control in Critically Ill Patients. (2009). *New England Journal of Medicine*, *360*(13), 1283–1297. doi: 10.1056/nejmoa0810625. https://www.nejm.org/doi/pdf/10.1056/NEJMoa0810625.

A. Kalinowski (✉)
Jefferson Health, Abington, PA, USA

J. Russell, N. S. Skolnik (eds.), *Top Articles in Primary Care*, https://doi.org/10.1007/978-3-031-25620-2_20

Design and Methods

- The investigators conducted a parallel-group, randomized, controlled trial involving adult medical and surgical patients admitted to the ICUs of 42 hospitals.
- Adults who were expected to require treatment in the ICU on 3 or more consecutive days were randomly assigned within 24 h of admission to the ICU to undergo either intensive glucose control (target blood glucose range of 81–108 mg/dL) or conventional glucose control (target blood glucose of 180 mg or less per deciliter).
- Control of blood glucose was achieved with the use of an intravenous infusion of insulin in saline.
- In the conventional glucose control group, insulin was administered if the blood glucose level exceeded 180 mg/dL. Insulin administration was reduced and then discontinued if the blood glucose level dropped below 144 mg/dL.
- The trial intervention was discontinued once the patient was eating or was discharged from the ICU but was resumed if the patient was readmitted to the ICU within 90 days.
- The trial intervention was discontinued permanently at the time of death or 90 days after randomization, whichever occurred first.
- The primary outcome measure was death from any cause within 90 days after randomization.
- Secondary outcome measures were survival time during the first 90 days, cause-specific death and durations of mechanical ventilation, renal-replacement therapy, and stays in the ICU and hospital.
- Tertiary outcomes were death from any cause within 28 days after randomization, place of death (ICU, hospital ward, or other), incidence of new organ failure, positive blood culture, receipt of red-cell transfusion, and volume of the transfusion.
- The primary outcome was also examined in six predefined pairs of subgroups: operative patients and nonoperative patients, patients with and those without diabetes, patients with and those without trauma, patients with and those without severe sepsis, patients treated and those not treated with corticosteroids, and patients whose APACHE II (a scoring system ranging from 0 to 71 developed to grade the severity of illness in acutely ill patients) score was 25 or more and those whose score was less than 25.
- A blood glucose level of 40 mg/dL (2.2 mmol/L) or less was considered a serious adverse event.

Results

- Study data was used from 6030 patients.
- The mean blood glucose level was significantly lower in the intensive-control group than in the conventional-control group (115 ± 18 vs. 144 ± 23 mg/dL).

- More patients in the conventional-control group received steroids, 34.6% vs. 31.7%. The most common indication for corticosteroid administration in both groups was the treatment of septic shock.
- Ninety days after randomization, 27.5% of patients in the intensive-control group had died, as compared with 24.9% of patients in the conventional-control group.
- Intensive glucose control increased mortality among adults in the ICU: A blood glucose target of 180 mg or less per deciliter resulted in lower mortality than did a target of 81–108 mg/dL.
- Deaths from cardiovascular causes were more common in the intensive-control group than in the conventional-control group.
- A similar number of patients developed new single or multiple organ failures in both groups.
- There was no significant difference between the two groups in the numbers of days of mechanical ventilation and renal-replacement therapy or in the rates of positive blood cultures and red-cell transfusion. There was no significant difference in mortality in comparisons of operative vs. non-operative patients, patients with and those without diabetes, those with or without severe sepsis, patients with an APACHE II score of 25 or more and those with a score of less than 25.
- Severe hypoglycemia was significantly more common with intensive glucose control.

Importance

Based on previous trials, intensive glucose control had been widely recommended prior to this study [1]. This study suggested that a goal of obtaining normoglycemia may be harmful to patients in an acutely ill state.

Bottom Line

Prior to this study, many professional organizations recommended tight glucose control for acutely ill patients. The investigators in this study conducted a parallel-group, randomized, controlled trial involving adult medical and surgical patients admitted to the ICU. Patients were randomized to a intensive glucose control group with a target blood glucose level of 81–108 or a conventional-control group with a target glucose range of 180 or less. Results of the study showed that intensive glucose control increased mortality among adults in the ICU.

Updates

In 2012, the NICE-SUGAR investigators examined the associations between moderate and severe hypoglycemia (blood glucose of 41–70 and ≤40 respectively) and death among 6026 critically ill patients in intensive care units. The intensively treated group had 10- to 15-fold greater rates of hypoglycemia, and hypoglycemia was strongly associated with mortality [2].

The current recommended glycemic targets in the Standards of Care of the American Diabetes Association is that, "Insulin therapy should be initiated for treatment of persistent hyperglycemia starting at a threshold of 180 mg/dL…Once insulin therapy is started, a target glucose range of 140–180 mg/dL is recommended for the majority of critically ill and noncritically ill patients. More stringent goals, such as 110–140 mg/dL, may be appropriate for selected patients if they can be achieved without significant hypoglycemia" [3].

References

1. Van den Berghe G, Wouters P, Weekers F, et al. Intensive insulin therapy in critically ill patients. N Engl J Med. 2001;345:1359–67.
2. NICE-SUGAR Study Investigators, et al. Hypoglycemia and risk of death in critically ill patients. N Engl J Med. 2012;367(12):1108–18. https://doi.org/10.1056/nejmoa1204942.
3. American Diabetes Association. 15. Diabetes care in the hospital: standards of medical care in diabetes—2021. Diabetes Care. 2021;44(Suppl-1):S211–20.

Chapter 21
Liraglutide and Cardiovascular Outcomes in Diabetes (LEADER)-2016

Gabriella Petrongolo

Background

The glucose lowering effects of hypoglycemic medications had been established for years, but the effect of these medications on macrovascular outcomes including MI, stoke, and CV mortality was not entirely clear. In 1998, the U.K. Prospective Diabetes Study (UKPDS) showed that intensive glucose lowering reduced microvascular complications in type 2 diabetes. It was not until 2008 that 10-year follow-up data from the UKPDS showed that treatment to reduce hyperglycemia also reduced macrovascular complications [1, 2]. In recognition of the importance of clear and direct disease oriented outcomes rather than just a "surrogate" outcome of A1c, in 2008 the FDA mandated CVOTs (Cardiovascular Outcome Trials) to be performed to establish cardiovascular safety for all new drugs brought to market [3]. The Liraglutide Effect and Action in Diabetes: Evaluation of Cardiovascular Outcomes Results (LEADER) trial was the first CVOT published for the GLP-1 Receptor Agonist class of medications.

Marso, S. P., Daniels, G. H., Brown-Frandsen, K., Kristensen, P., Mann, J. F., Nauck, M. A., Nissen, S. E., Pocock, S., Poulter, N. R., Ravn, L. S., Steinberg, W. M., Stockner, M., Zinman, B., Bergenstal, R. M., Buse, J. B., LEADER Steering Committee, & LEADER Trial Investigators (2016). Liraglutide and Cardiovascular Outcomes in Type 2 Diabetes. The New England Journal of Medicine, 375(4), 311–322. https://doi.org/10.1056/NEJMoa1603827.
Hyperlink to PDF: https://pubmed.ncbi.nlm.nih.gov/27295427/.

G. Petrongolo (✉)
Jefferson Health, Abington, PA, USA
e-mail: gabriella.petrongolo@jefferson.edu

J. Russell, N. S. Skolnik (eds.), *Top Articles in Primary Care*,
https://doi.org/10.1007/978-3-031-25620-2_21

Objective

The LEADER trial was initiated to evaluate the effects of liraglutide on long-term cardiovascular outcomes in those with type 2 diabetes mellitus. The primary outcome studied was death from cardiovascular cause, nonfatal myocardial infarction, or nonfatal stroke. The hypothesis was that liraglutide would be noninferior to placebo.

Design and Methods

- The trial was a placebo-controlled and double-blinded study. Participants were randomly assigned to receive either 1.8 mg subcutaneous liraglutide daily or 1.8 mg subcutaneous placebo daily.
- Participants were recruited from 410 sites across 32 countries. All participants were diagnosed with type 2 diabetes mellitus with an HgA1c over 7.0%. They were over 50 years of age with known cardiovascular disease, or over 60 years of age with cardiovascular risk factors.
- Exclusion criteria included diagnosis of type 1 diabetes mellitus, previous use of GLP-1 receptor agonist, DDP-4 inhibitor, or rapid acting insulin class medications, those with history or family history of multiple endocrine neoplasia type 2, medullary thyroid cancer, or acute coronary or cardiovascular events within 2 weeks of study screening.
- Participant follow-up occurred at months 1, 3, 6, and then every 6 months until months 42–60 after initiation of trial.
- Participants who did not reach the recommended glycemic goal of a HgA1c below 7.0% during participation were permitted to start additional antihyperglycemic medications during trial, excluding GLP-1 receptor agonist, DPP-4 inhibitors, or pramlintide.
- Primary outcomes evaluated included death from cardiovascular cause, nonfatal myocardial infarction, or nonfatal stroke. Other exploratory outcomes included need for coronary revascularization, hospitalization for heart failure or unstable angina, death from any cause, nephropathy, retinopathy, neoplasm, and pancreatitis.

Results

- The primary outcome studied, the rate of first occurrence of death from cardiovascular cause, nonfatal myocardial infarction, and nonfatal stroke, occurred in a statistically significant fewer number of participants in the liraglutide group than in the placebo group (hazard ratio of 0.87; $P < 0.001$ for noninferiority; $P = 0.01$ for superiority).

- Other statistically significant findings included lower cardiovascular mortallity (hazard ratio, 0.78; $P = 0.007$), fewer incidences of death from any cause (hazard ratio, 0.85; $P = 0.02$).
- The rates of nonfatal myocardial infarction, nonfatal stroke, and hospitalization for heart failure were nonsignificantly lower in the liraglutide group than in the placebo group.
- There was also a lower incidence of nephropathy lower rate of nephropathy events in the liraglutide group (hazard ratio, 0.78; $P = 0.003$)
- The most-experienced adverse drug reactions in the liraglutide group were gastrointestinal-related and included nausea, vomiting, diarrhea, decreased appetite, abdominal discomfort and abdominal pain. There was a statistically significant increased incidence of acute gallstone disease in the liraglutide group when compared to placebo.

Importance

This large, multi-center, double-blinded study was performed to understand more about the effects of GLP-1 receptor agonists on long-term cardiovascular outcomes in individuals with type 2 diabetes mellitus. The study was the first CVOT in the GLP-1 RA class of medications that showed that beyond just blood glucose control, the GLP-1 RA class of medications improve cardiovascular outcomes.

Updates

This was the first of the CVOTs in the GLP-1 RA class that showed a positive outcome on cardiovascular endpoints. Since then the CVOTs for dulaglutide (REWIND trial) and semaglutide (SUSTAIN) have also shown cardiovascular benefit [4, 5].

Bottom Line

The results of the CVOTs for both the SGLT-2 inhibitor and the GLP-1 RA classes of medicine have led to changes in the standards of care by the American Diabetes Association for managing diabetes, with the recommendations now for people with established vascular disease or at high risk of vascular disease to preferential be on a GLP-1 RA or an SGLT-2 inhibitor [6].

References

1. UK Prospective Diabetes Study Group. Intensive blood-glucose control with sulphonylureas or insulin compared with conventional treatment and risk of complications in patients with type 2 diabetes (UKPDS 33). Lancet. 1998;352:837–53.
2. Holman RR, Paul SK, Bethel MA, Matthews DR, Neil HA. 10-year follow-up of intensive glucose control in type 2 diabetes. N Engl J Med. 2008;359:1577–89.
3. U.S. Food and Drug Administration. Guidance for industry: diabetes mellitus: evaluating cardiovascular risk in new antidiabetic therapies to treat type 2 diabetes. https://wayback.archive-it.org/7993/20190917012500/https://www.fda.gov/media/71297/download.
4. Gerstein HC, Colhoun HM, Dagenais GR, et al. REWIND Investigators. Dulaglutide and cardiovascular outcomes in type 2 diabetes (REWIND): a double-blind, randomised placebo-controlled trial. Lancet. 2019;394:121–30.
5. Marso SP, Bain SC, Consoli A, et al. SUSTAIN-6 Investigators. Semaglutide and cardiovascular outcomes in patients with type 2 diabetes. N Engl J Med. 2016;375:1834–44.
6. Standards of care in diabetes 2022. Diabetes Care. 2022;45(Suppl 1):1–259.

Part IV
Hypertension

Margot Boigon

Chapter 22
Systolic Hypertension in the Elderly (SHEP)-1991

Bryce Eng and Meera Shah

Background

Isolated systolic hypertension (ISH) has high prevalence in those older than 65, roughly 30%, and accounts for the majority of uncontrolled hypertension cases, 80%, compared to diastolic hypertension [1, 2]. This prevalence results from aging's increased arterial wall stiffness coupled with chronic disease changes from inflammation and oxidative stress. Prior studies such as the Framingham Heart Study had begun establishing greater concern for systolic hypertension over diastolic hypertension in the elderly because ISH is a stronger predictor of coronary artery disease and worse cardiovascular outcomes [2, 3]. This led to studies such as SHEP which postulated that treatment of ISH would improve cardiovascular outcomes.

Objective

- The primary objective of the SHEP trial was to investigate whether treatment of isolated systolic hypertension leads to a reduction in total stroke outcomes.
- Secondary outcomes included cardiac events, morbidity, and mortality.

SHEP Cooperative Research Group. (1991). Prevention of stroke by antihypertensive drug treatment in older persons with isolated systolic hypertension. Jama, 265, 3255-3264.
Hyperlink to PDF: http://files.constantcontact.com/12c78154501/1b6cd57d-534a-4401-a755-c3a75e7662b0.pdf.

B. Eng (✉) · M. Shah
Jefferson Health, Abington, PA, USA
e-mail: bryce.eng@jefferson.edu; meera.shah@jefferson.edu

J. Russell, N. S. Skolnik (eds.), *Top Articles in Primary Care*,
https://doi.org/10.1007/978-3-031-25620-2_22

Design and Methods

- Double-blind randomized, placebo-controlled trial involving 4735 men and women aged 60 years and older with systolic blood pressure (SBP) ≥160 mmHg and diastolic blood pressure (DBP) <90 mmHg.
- Mean age was 72 years old. Fifty-seven percent were women and 14% were African American.
- Active treatment group had a SBP goal reduction of 20 mmHg, with the first medication administered chlorthalidone 12.5 mg daily titrated up to 25 mg daily followed by atenolol 25 mg daily or reserpine 0.05 mg daily if goal SBP was not yet met.
- Participants were unblinded and given known antihypertensive treatment if escape criteria were met (single visit SBP >240 mmHg or single visit DBP >115 mmHg; sustained SBP >220 mmHg or sustained DBP >90 mmHg).
- Patients with atrial fibrillation, major cardiovascular disease (history of myocardial infarction, heart failure, coronary artery bypass), renal failure, alcoholic liver disease, and cancer were excluded.
- Blood pressure checks were done at quarterly visits and average follow-up period was 4.5 years.
- Analysis was intention-to-treat.

Results

- Active treatment group had an average blood pressure decrease of 26/9 and the placebo group of 15/4.
- Nearly half of the active treatment group required only chlorthalidone and over two-thirds received chlorthalidone and/or a second agent.
- At the 5 year visit, 65% of participants in the active group and 40% from the placebo group met their targeted goal of SBP reduction.
- Significant outcomes: 36% reduction in total stroke incidence and 27% decrease in nonfatal myocardial infarction and coronary death incidence.
- Nonsignificant outcomes: 32% reduction in cardiovascular events and 13% reduction in mortality. No increase in dementia or depression rates.

Importance

The SHEP trial set a precedent for addressing isolated systolic hypertension in the elderly and showed that with a goal SBP of less than 160 mmHg, a simple antihypertensive regimen could improve cardiovascular outcomes without major adverse effects. The SHEP trial would be followed by future studies such as the HYVET

Table 22.1 Guideline recommendations for systolic blood pressure control in the elderly

	ACP/AAFP (2017) [4]	AHA/ACC (2017) [5]
Drug initiation SBP threshold for patients >60 years old without history of CVD, CKD, or diabetes mellitus	150	140

trial and SPRINT trial which have further sought to clarify goal antihypertensive threshold and regimen for the geriatric population. Since SHEP's publication, societal guidelines have agreed that systolic hypertension in the elderly should be treated but most recent updates from the ACP/AAFP [4] and AHA/ACC [5] differ in goal SBP threshold recommendations due to differing opinions about the risks/benefits of aggressive management (Table 22.1)

Updates

- The Syst-Eur trial (1997) and HYVET trial (2008) further supported the SHEP trial's findings by showing similar significant reduction in strokes and certain cardiac endpoints [6, 7].
- With evidence from meta-analyses [8, 9], the AHA has recommended that blood pressure reduction has a greater effect than choosing a specific drug class in improving cardiovascular outcomes [5].
- The SPRINT trial (2015) showed significantly lower cardiovascular composite primary endpoint rates and mortality for goal SBP <120 mmHg compared to <140 mmHg with similar results in its subgroup for those ≥75 years old [10]. This trial would inform the recent AHA/ACC guidelines [5].

Bottom Line

- Systolic hypertension ≥150 mmHg in the elderly should be treated with antihypertensives as this intervention reduces the risk of stroke and other cardiovascular events.

References

1. Burt VL, Whelton P, Roccella EJ, Brown C, Cutler JA, Higgins M, et al. Prevalence of hypertension in the US adult population: results from the Third National Health and Nutrition Examination Survey, 1988-1991. Hypertension. 1995;25(3):305–13.
2. Franklin SS, Gustin W IV, Wong ND, Larson MG, Weber MA, Kannel WB, Levy D. Hemodynamic patterns of age-related changes in blood pressure: the Framingham Heart Study. Circulation. 1997;96(1):308–15.

3. Izzo JL Jr, Levy D, Black HR. Importance of systolic blood pressure in older Americans. Hypertension. 2000;35(5):1021–4.
4. Qaseem A, Wilt TJ, Rich R, Humphrey LL, Frost J, Forciea MA, Clinical Guidelines Committee of the American College of Physicians and the Commission on Health of the Public and Science of the American Academy of Family Physicians. Pharmacologic treatment of hypertension in adults aged 60 years or older to higher versus lower blood pressure targets: a clinical practice guideline from the American College of Physicians and the American Academy of Family Physicians. Ann Intern Med. 2017;166(6):430–7.
5. Whelton PK, Carey RM, Aronow WS, Casey DE, Collins KJ, Dennison Himmelfarb C, et al. 2017 ACC/AHA/AAPA/ABC/ACPM/AGS/APhA/ASH/ASPC/NMA/PCNA guideline for the prevention, detection, evaluation, and management of high blood pressure in adults: a report of the American College of Cardiology/American Heart Association Task Force on Clinical Practice Guidelines. J Am Coll Cardiol. 2018;71(19):e127–248.
6. Staessen JA, Fagard R, Thijs L, Celis H, Arabidze GG, Birkenhäger WH, et al. Randomised double-blind comparison of placebo and active treatment for older patients with isolated systolic hypertension. Lancet. 1997;350(9080):757–64.
7. Beckett NS, Peters R, Fletcher AE, Staessen JA, Liu L, Dumitrascu D, et al. Treatment of hypertension in patients 80 years of age or older. N Engl J Med. 2008;358(18):1887–98.
8. Trialists' Collaboration, B. P. L. T. Effects of different regimens to lower blood pressure on major cardiovascular events in older and younger adults: meta-analysis of randomised trials. Br Med J. 2008;336(7653):1121–3.
9. Law M, Morris JK, Wald N. Use of blood pressure lowering drugs in the prevention of cardiovascular disease: meta-analysis of 147 randomised trials in the context of expectations from prospective epidemiological studies. Br Med J. 2009;338:b1665.
10. SPRINT Research Group. Final report of a trial of intensive versus standard blood-pressure control. N Engl J Med. 2021;384(20):1921–30.

Chapter 23
Dietary Patterns in Hypertension (DASH)-1997

Morgan Katz

Background

Hypertension is a very common problem in the USA. Hypertension accounted for more CVD than any other modifiable cardiovascular disease risk factor [1]. Prior to the DASH study, efforts to reduce hypertension had been mostly focused on pharmacologic intervention. Non-pharmacologic interventions such as weight loss, decreased dietary sodium, and decreased alcohol assumption had been studied, but effects of dietary patterns had not yet been fully studied.

Objective

The Dietary Approaches to Stop Hypertension (DASH) trial's goal was to study the effects of dietary patterns on treating and preventing hypertension. The study aimed to look at patterns in diet, rather than individual nutrients in order to test the combined effect of nutrients that occur together in foods.

Appel LJ, Moore TJ, Obarzanek E, et al. *A clinical trial of the effects of dietary patterns on blood pressure.* DASH Collaborative Research Group. N Engl J Med 1997; 336:1117. https://www.nejm.org/doi/pdf/10.1056/NEJM199704173361601.

M. Katz (✉)
Jefferson Health, Abington, PA, USA

Primary Care, ChristianaCare, Newark, USA

J. Russell, N. S. Skolnik (eds.), *Top Articles in Primary Care*,
https://doi.org/10.1007/978-3-031-25620-2_23

Design and Methods

- 459 patients 22 years and older of age with SBP >160 mmHg and DBP 80–95 mmHg were randomized to 3 different diets: a control diet, a diet rich in fruits and vegetables, and a diet rich in fruits and vegetables and low-fat diary products along with foods low in saturated and total fat.
- Persons with medication-treated hypertension could enroll if they met the inclusion criteria for blood pressure after supervised withdrawal of medication.
- Exclusion criteria—poorly controlled diabetes; hyperlipidemia; a cardiovascular event within the previous 6 months; chronic diseases that might interfere with participation; pregnancy or lactation; BMI >35; the use of medications that affect blood pressure; unwillingness to stop taking vitamin and mineral supplements or antacids containing magnesium or calcium; CKD, excessive alcohol intake.
- All participants were advised to reduce sodium intake and alcohol consumption
- For the first 3 weeks, subjects all ate a control diet which was low in fruits, vegetables, and dairy products
- For the following 8 weeks, they were monitored following their assigned diets, while sodium intake and body weight were maintained at constant levels

Results

- Participants in the fruit and diet rich in fruits and vegetables reduced BP by 2.8/1.1 mmHg over control, while the combination diet reduced BP by 5.5/3.0 mmHg over control.

Importance

The DASH diet shows the importance and effect of dietary intervention in hypertension. The reduction in BP shown in the study is similar to that observed in trials of drug monotherapy for mild hypertension. This is one of the important studies that have influenced guidelines to include dietary advice as a part of initial lifestyle modification for initial treatment or in addition to pharmacologic treatment, depending upon the stage of hypertension, for patients diagnosed with hypertension.

Updates

- The DASH diet has been found to also improve insulin sensitivity along with other metabolic abnormalities [2]

Bottom Line

- The DASH diet (a diet rich in fruit, vegetables, and low fat dairy foods) can substantially lower blood pressure and is effective in both treating and preventing hypertension.

References

1. Whelton PK, et al. 2017 ACC/AHA/AAPA/ABC/ACPM/AGS/APhA/ASH/ASPC/NMA/PCNA guideline for the prevention, detection, evaluation, and management of high blood pressure in adults: a report of the American College of Cardiology/American Heart Association Task Force on clinical practice guidelines. J Am Coll Cardiol. 2018;71:e127–248.
2. Hinderliter AL, Babyak MA, Sherwood A, et al. The DASH diet and insulin sensitivity. Curr Hypertens Rep. 2011;13:67–73. https://doi.org/10.1007/s11906-010-0168-5.

Chapter 24
Comparison of Medications for Hypertension (ALLHAT)-2002

Nathaniel Rosal

Background

Hypertension is strongly associated with increased cardiovascular events if left uncontrolled. By the end of the twentieth century, many antihypertensive medications were widely available and proven to be efficacious. However, their effects on different cardiovascular events were uncertain. Newer agents, including ACE inhibitors, calcium channel blockers (CCBs), and alpha-adrenergic blockers, had not been compared to the older agents.

Objective

- To compare the difference in incidence of cardiovascular disease (CVD) events of CCBs, ACE inhibitors, and alpha-adrenergic blockers compared to thiazide diuretics.

ALLHAT Officers and Coordinators for the ALLHAT Collaborative Research Group. The Antihypertensive and Lipid-Lowering Treatment to Prevent Heart Attack Trial (2002). Major outcomes in high-risk hypertensive patients randomized to angiotensin-converting enzyme inhibitor or calcium channel blocker vs diuretic: The Antihypertensive and Lipid-Lowering Treatment to Prevent Heart Attack Trial (ALLHAT). JAMA, 288(23), 2981–2997. https://doi.org/10.1001/jama.288.23.2981.
Hyperlink to PDF: https://jamanetwork.com/journals/jama/fullarticle/195626.

N. Rosal (✉)
Jefferson Health, Abington, PA, USA
e-mail: Nathaniel.Rosal@jefferson.edu

J. Russell, N. S. Skolnik (eds.), *Top Articles in Primary Care*,
https://doi.org/10.1007/978-3-031-25620-2_24

Design and Methods

- Study design: randomized, double blinded, active-controlled, clinical trial.
- Setting: multicenter (623 North American centers).
- Participants: 33,357 participants aged 55 or older with a diagnosis of hypertension and at least one other coronary heart disease risk factor.
- Primary outcome: combined fatal coronary heart disease (CHD) or nonfatal myocardial infarction.
- Secondary outcomes: all-cause mortality, stroke, combined CHD (primary outcome, revascularization, or angina requiring hospitalization) and combined CVD (combined CHD, stroke, treated angina not requiring hospitalization, heart failure, and PAD).
- Calcium channel blockers were represented by amlodipine, ACE inhibitors were represented by lisinopril, alpha-adrenergic blockers were represented by doxazosin, and thiazide diuretics were represented by chlorthalidone.

Results

- Five-year systolic blood pressures were higher in the amlodipine and lisinopril groups when compared to the chlorthalidone group.
- Amlodipine had a higher 6-year rate of heart failure when compared to chlorthalidone.
- Lisinopril had a higher 6-year rate of combined, stroke, and heart failure when compared to chlorthalidone.
- The Doxazosin arm was terminated early due to an increase in the incidence of heart failure.
- All-cause mortality did not differ between the groups.

Importance

Leading up to the release of the ALLHAT Trial, calcium channel blockers, ACE inhibitors, and alpha-adrenergic blockers were proven useful for hypertension management but whether they were superior to thiazide diuretics was unknown. This trial compared these newer agents to the older class of thiazides. Following ALLHAT, alpha-blockers were no longer considered a first-line medication for the treatment of hypertension. Chlorthalidone, calcium channel blockers, and ACE-inhibitors were shown to have similar effects on mortality, with different effects on heart failure and stroke. These findings were consistent with prior trials (the authors cite the EWPHE trial and INSIGHT trial).

Updates

- A 2006 post-trial follow-up study investigated patients in the ALLHAT trial who developed new onset heart failure (HF). All-cause mortality rates were similar when comparing anti-hypertensive medication groups, but risk of death was high for patients with HF in both groups [1].
- ALLHAT sparked a debate regarding the choice of thiazide diuretic. While chlorthalidone was the thiazide used in this trial, hydrochlorothiazide was the most prescribed in this class (possibly due to price and availability) [2]. This resulted in many studies investigating the efficacy and safety profile between these two drugs, and the results were conflicting. Fifteen years following the release of ALLHAT, the 2017 American College of Cardiology/American Heart Association hypertension guidelines recommended chlorthalidone over hydrochlorothiazide as the preferred thiazide diuretic for essential hypertension [3].
- A 2020 observational comparative cohort study involving 730,225 patients found no significant difference between risk of MI, heart failure, or stroke in patients being treated with hydrochlorothiazide versus patients being treated with chlorthalidone [4].

Bottom Line

- Chlorthalidone was similar to lisinopril and amlodipine in prevention of CAD and nonfatal MI. Notably it had a lower incidence of heart failure and led to better blood pressure control. Alpha-blockers are no longer considered a first-line medication for the treatment of hypertension.
- Based on ALLHAT, as well as other trials, the current the 2017 American College of Cardiology/American Heart Association hypertension guidelines recommend initial first-line therapy for stage 1 hypertension includes thiazide diuretics, CCBs, and ACE inhibitors or ARBs.

References

1. Piller LB, Baraniuk S, Simpson LM, Cushman WC, Massie BM, Einhorn PT, Oparil S, Ford CE, Graumlich JF, Dart RA, Parish DC, Retta TM, Cuyjet AB, Jafri SZ, Furberg CD, Saklayen MG, Thadani U, Probstfield JL, Davis BR, ALLHAT Collaborative Research Group. Long-term follow-up of participants with heart failure in the antihypertensive and lipid-lowering treatment to prevent heart attack trial (ALLHAT). Circulation. 2011;124(17):1811–8. https://doi.org/10.1161/CIRCULATIONAHA.110.012575.
2. Kaplan NM. The choice of thiazide diuretics: why chlorthalidone may replace hydrochlorothiazide. Hypertension. 2009;54(5):951–3. https://doi.org/10.1161/HYPERTENSIONAHA.109.135061.

3. Whelton PK, Carey RM, Aronow WS, Casey DE Jr, Collins KJ, Dennison Himmelfarb C, DePalma SM, Gidding S, Jamerson KA, Jones DW, MacLaughlin EJ, Muntner P, Ovbiagele B, Smith SC Jr, Spencer CC, Stafford RS, Taler SJ, Thomas RJ, Williams KA Sr, Williamson JD, Wright JT Jr. 2017 ACC/AHA/AAPA/ABC/ACPM/AGS/APhA/ASH/ASPC/NMA/PCNA guideline for the prevention, detection, evaluation, and management of high blood pressure in adults: executive summary: a report of the American College of Cardiology/American Heart Association Task Force on Clinical Practice Guidelines. Circulation. 2018;138(17):e426–83. https://doi.org/10.1161/CIR.0000000000000597.
4. Hripcsak G, Suchard MA, Shea S, et al. Comparison of cardiovascular and safety outcomes of chlorthalidone vs hydrochlorothiazide to treat hypertension. JAMA Intern Med. 2020;180(4):542–51. https://doi.org/10.1001/jamainternmed.2019.7454.

Chapter 25
Intensive Versus Standard Blood Pressure Control (SPRINT)-2015

Alyssa J. Style

Background

Hypertension is the most common disease seen in primary care [1] and affects 1 billion adults around the world. Systolic blood pressure (SBP) is a risk factor for coronary events, stroke, heart failure, and end-stage renal disease. While we know that treating hypertension reduces cardiovascular disease, the extent to which SBP should be lowered to best achieve this benefit had not yet been determined.

Objective

- To determine if there is a cardiovascular and overall mortality benefit associated with a SBP target <120 mm Hg compared to <140 mm Hg in adults without diabetes.

SPRINT Research Group. (2015). A Randomized Trial of Intensive versus Standard Blood-Pressure Control. New England Journal of Medicine, 373(22), 2103–2116. doi: 10.1056/nejmoa1511939
Hyperlink to PDF: https://www.nejm.org/doi/pdf/10.1056/NEJMoa1511939

A. J. Style (✉)
Jefferson Health, Abington, PA, USA

J. Russell, N. S. Skolnik (eds.), *Top Articles in Primary Care*,
https://doi.org/10.1007/978-3-031-25620-2_25

Design and Methods

- Randomized, controlled, open label trial with intention to treat analysis
- Conducted at 102 clinical sites in the USA, $n = 9250$ participants
- Inclusion criteria: ≥50 years old, SBP between 130 and 180 mm Hg, increased risk of cardiovascular events defined as:
  - Clinical or subclinical cardiovascular disease not including stroke
  - Chronic kidney disease (eGFR 20–59 ml per minute per 1.73 m^2), excluding polycystic kidney disease
  - 10-year cardiovascular risk of ≥15% based on Framingham risk score
  - ≥75 years old
- Exclusion criteria: diabetes mellitus, prior stroke
- Primary endpoints: myocardial infarction, acute coronary syndrome not resulting in myocardial infarction, stroke, acute decompensated heart failure, or death from cardiovascular causes
- Secondary endpoint: all-cause mortality
- 2 treatment groups:
  - Standard treatment group: systolic blood pressure target 135–139 mm Hg
  - Intensive treatment group: systolic blood pressure target <120 mm Hg
- Participants were monitored monthly for 3 months and then at 3 month intervals. Medications were adjusted based on a mean of three blood pressure measurements obtained during an office visit.
- Serious adverse events (fatal or life-threatening, resulting in disability, requiring prolonged hospitalization, requiring medical or surgical intervention) were monitored as well as additional adverse events that required an emergency room evaluation. This included hypotension, syncope, injurious falls, electrolyte abnormalities, bradycardia, and acute kidney injury.

Results

- Lowering the SBP target from <140 to <120 mm Hg resulted in lower rates of fatal and nonfatal cardiovascular events and death from any cause in adults without diabetes.
- Number needed to treat
  - Prevent a primary outcome event: 61
  - Death from any cause: 90
  - Death from cardiovascular causes: 172
- Study ended early after 3.26 years due to significant benefit of intervention.
- More adverse events occurred in the intensive treatment group (38.3%) when compared to the standard treatment group (37.1%).

- Acute kidney injury occurred more frequently in the intensive treatment group in those without chronic kidney disease. There was no difference in renal function between treatment groups in those with chronic kidney disease.

Importance

The SPRINT trial played an important role in altering the management of hypertension in adults without diabetes who are at high risk of cardiovascular events. Lowering the SBP target will increase the number of individuals treated for hypertension. This study demonstrated that a SBP target of <120 mmHg versus <140 mm Hg decreases cardiovascular disease and all-cause mortality.

Updates

- The American College of Cardiology (ACC) and American Heart Association (AHA) redefined hypertension as ≥130/80 mm Hg [2].
- The American Academy of Family Physicians did not endorse the new ACC/AHA guideline. They continue to support the 2014 Evidence-Based Guideline for the Management of High Blood Pressure in Adults (JNC-8) that recommends a blood pressure target <140/90 mm Hg for individuals less than 60 years old [3].

Bottom Line

- In adults without diabetes, lowering the SBP target from <140 mm Hg to <120 mm Hg resulted in lower rates of fatal and nonfatal cardiovascular events and death from any cause.

References

1. James PA. 2014 guideline for management of high blood pressure. 2014. Retrieved November 11, 2019, from https://jamanetwork.com/journals/jama/fullarticle/1791497
2. 2017 guideline for high blood pressure in adults. 2018. Retrieved November 10, 2019, from https://www.acc.org/latest in cardiology/ten-points-to-remember/2017/11/09/11/41/2017-guideline-for-high-blood-pressure-in-adults.
3. LeFevre M. ACC/AHA hypertension guideline: what is new? What do we do? 2018. Retrieved November 10, 2019, from https://www.aafp.org/afp/2018/0315/p372.html.

Chapter 26
Intensive BP Control in Older Patients (STEP)-2021

Stephanie Tzarnas

Background

Cardiovascular disease remains the leading cause of death worldwide among populations. Hypertension is the most common risk factor for cardiovascular disease [1]. In addition, hypertension remains the most modifiable risk factor for preventable disease, specifically, cardiovascular disease. Hypertension more commonly affects individuals over the age of 60 and its prevalence increases with age [2]. Guideline based recommendations for blood pressure targets in older hypertensive patients can be inconsistent [3]. The STEP (Strategy of Blood Pressure Intervention in the Elderly Hypertensive Patients) trial assesses the impact on intensive versus standard blood pressure control in the reduction of cardiovascular risk.

Objective

- To compare the reduction of cardiovascular risk between intensive treatment of blood pressure control to standard treatment of blood pressure control

Zhang, Weili, et al, Trial of Intensive Blood-Pressure Control in Older Patients with Hypertension. N Engl J Med 2021; 385, 1268–1279.
Article PDF: https://www.nejm.org/doi/pdf/10.1056/NEJMoa2111437?articleTools=true

S. Tzarnas (✉)
Jefferson Health, Abington, PA, USA
e-mail: Stephanie.Tzarnas@jefferson.edu

J. Russell, N. S. Skolnik (eds.), *Top Articles in Primary Care*, https://doi.org/10.1007/978-3-031-25620-2_26

Design and Methods

- The study included just over 8500 Chinese patients aged 60–80 years old with a diagnosis of hypertension in a prospective, multi-center, randomized controlled trial with the primary endpoint of cardiovascular risk—specifically, a primary outcome composite of stroke, acute coronary syndrome, acute decompensated heart failure, coronary revascularization, atrial fibrillation, or death from cardiovascular causes.
- Patients were randomly assigned to the intensive treatment group or to the standard treatment group.
  - Intensive treatment group: systolic blood pressure target of 110 to <130 mm Hg
  - Standard treatment group: systolic blood pressure target of 130 to <150 mm Hg
- All patients were scheduled for follow-up office visits every 3 months and recorded home blood pressure readings via a smart phone application every week.
- Cardiovascular disease risk was estimated using the Framingham Risk Score.
- Data was evaluated with an intention to treat analysis.

Results

- The mean systolic blood pressure of the intensive treatment group was 127.5 mm Hg at 1 year follow-up compared to the mean systolic blood pressure of 135.3 mm Hg in the standard treatment group.
- The intensive treatment group had a significantly lower incidence (3.5%) of primary outcome events at two consecutive time points over a follow-up period of 3 years. The data and safety monitoring committee recommended that the trial be stopped early since there was a clear reduction of cardiovascular risk in the intensive treatment group.
- The intensive treatment group also had lower incidences of individual primary outcome events (stroke, acute coronary syndrome, acute decompensated heart failure, coronary revascularization, atrial fibrillation, or death from cardiovascular causes) compared to the standard treatment group.
- The incidence of hypotension was significantly higher in the intensive treatment group; however, the incidence of dizziness, syncope, and fracture did not differ significantly between the two treatment groups.

Importance

Previous trials have shown that a reduction in overall systolic blood pressure resulted in decreased cardiovascular risk. The SPRINT trial showed a blood pressure goal of less than a systolic of 120 mmHg vs. systolic BP < 140 led to a decrease in the composite cardiovascular endpoint in individuals with cardiovascular disease or elevated cardiovascular risk of >15% 10-year risk [4]. Changing of the blood pressure target from the traditional goal of <140 mmHg has been controversial, as the recommendations were based on one trial and there have been concerns raised on the generalization of the blood pressure assessment method used in the SPRINT trial. The STEP trial corroborated the results of the SPRINT trial, and so will likely have a major role in determining a systolic blood pressure goal in older patients. Specifically, a reduction in the systolic blood pressure to less than 130 mm Hg resulted in decreased cardiovascular risk in older hypertensive Chinese patients.

The STEP trial was one of the first to use home blood pressure monitoring in addition to office blood pressure readings in data collection. The difference between systolic blood pressure at home versus in the office was consistent between treatment groups. This provided not only realistic blood pressure readings but also more accurately represented long term variations in blood pressure. In addition, home blood pressure readings were easier for patients to obtain.

Bottom Line

- Aggressive systolic blood pressure management in older adults with a systolic BP goal of <130 mm Hg results in a lower incidence of cardiovascular events and leads to decreased cardiovascular risk.

References

1. Kjeldsen SE. Hypertension and cardiovascular risk: general aspects. Pharmacol Res. 2018;129:95–9. https://doi.org/10.1016/j.phrs.2017.11.003.
2. Wu CY, Hu HY, Chou YJ, Huang N, Chou YC, Li CP. High blood pressure and all-cause and cardiovascular disease mortalities in community-dwelling older adults. Medicine. 2015;94(47):e2160. https://doi.org/10.1097/MD.0000000000002160.
3. Saiz LC, Gorricho J, Garjón J, Celaya MC, Erviti J, Leache L. Blood pressure targets for the treatment of people with hypertension and cardiovascular disease. Cochrane Database Syst Rev. 2020;9(9):CD010315. https://doi.org/10.1002/14651858.CD010315.pub4.
4. SPRINT Research Group. A randomized trial of intensive versus standard blood-pressure control. N Engl J Med. 2015;373(22):2103–16. https://doi.org/10.1056/nejmoa1511939.

Part V
Infectious Disease

John Russell

Chapter 27
Penicillin for Strep Throat to Reduce Rheumatic Heart Disease-1950

Mathew Clark

Background

Rheumatic fever was a feared and fairly common disease in the early 1900s. By the 1940s, it was understood that rheumatic fever was related to streptococcal infection, and streptococcal infection had been shown to respond to antibiotics "miracle drugs", which had only recently become available. At the time of this study, however, no one had connected these dots: Could treatment with antibiotics, once a patient had a streptococcal illness, prevent rheumatic fever?

Objective

To determine, in a population with acute streptococcal pharyngitis, whether treatment with penicillin prevented the subsequent development of rheumatic fever.

Denny FW, Wannamaker LW, Brink WR, et. al. (1950) Prevention of rheumatic fever; treatment of the preceding Streptococcic infection. JAMA 143(2)151 3.
https://jamanetwork.com/journals/jama/fullarticle/291372

M. Clark (✉)
Jefferson Health, Abington, PA, USA
e-mail: mathew.clark@jefferson.edu

J. Russell, N. S. Skolnik (eds.), *Top Articles in Primary Care*,
https://doi.org/10.1007/978-3-031-25620-2_27

Design and Methods

- 1634 soldiers at an army base in Wyoming, who were diagnosed clinically with strep pharyngitis.
- Randomized to receive penicillin injections—300,00 units, 2 or 3 doses, 2 days apart—vs no antibiotics.
- Participants had throat cultures, as well as acute and convalescent ASO titers.
- Assessed for rheumatic fever 3–4 weeks after infection, using Jones criteria [1]

Results

- Roughly 800 patients in each group
- Untreated group had 23 cases of rheumatic fever (2%)
- Treated group had only 4 cases of rheumatic fever (0.5%)

Importance

This study, done during the first decade of widespread antibiotic availability, clarified the role of penicillin in helping to eradicate streptococcal infection from the pharynx, and showed that timely treatment dramatically reduced the chance of developing acute rheumatic fever.

It is interesting to read this study through the lens of the subsequent decades of experience with antibiotics and the evolution of public health thinking. We have seen acute rheumatic fever became extremely rare, and deaths from this condition—7 per 100,000 in 1900—essentially no longer occur in the USA. Very little of this change appears to be due to the use of antibiotics; a graph of rheumatic fever and related deaths shows a steady downward curve, approaching zero, with almost no inflection before or after the introduction of penicillin. So the case for antibiotic treatment of strep pharyngitis has become less compelling, at the same time that concerns about antibiotic overuse, development of resistance, and potential side effects have grown. Nevertheless, this study continues to inform and drive our current approach to adults who present with acute pharyngitis.

Bottom Line

This was the first study to clearly link the treatment of streptococcal pharyngitis, using penicillin, with significantly decreasing the risk of subsequent rheumatic fever. Although many of the conditions which existed at the time of this study may no longer apply, it continues to drive our practice patterns, 72 years later.

Reference

1. Jones TD. The diagnosis of rheumatic fever. JAMA. 1944;126:481.

Chapter 28
CDC's Report of First Cases of AIDS in US-1981

Anne Sprogell and John Russell

Background

Pneumocystis carinii pneumonia (PCP), now known as *Pneumocystis jirovecii* pneumonia (PJP) is almost exclusively seen in patients who are severely immunocompromised. What was startling about these cases was that the 5 men were previously healthy and had no obvious common sick contacts. PCP was first discovered in 1955. It was exclusively seen in patients with immunodeficiencies. A paper in 1974 in Annals of Internal Medicine [1] described only 194 cases reported to the CDC over a 3 year period of time. From 1967 on, The CDC was the sole provider of pentamidine, which at the time was the only available treatment for PCP and not yet available in the USA.

Objective

To highlight a pattern of young men in Los Angeles with PJP, CMV, and candida mucosal infection.

Pneumocystis Pneumonia -- Los Angeles. (n.d.). Retrieved from https://www.cdc.gov/mmwr/preview/mmwrhtml/00043494.htm.

A. Sprogell (✉) · J. Russell
Jefferson Health, Abington, PA, USA
e-mail: john.russell@jefferson.edu

J. Russell, N. S. Skolnik (eds.), *Top Articles in Primary Care*,
https://doi.org/10.1007/978-3-031-25620-2_28

Importance

After these case reports were published, similar cases were noted in New York. Employees at the CDC who dispensed the treatment for PJP saw a pattern marking the beginning of the AIDS epidemic and the public health efforts to define, monitor, prevent, and eventually treat it.

Updates

PJP, CMV, and candidal mucosal infections, along with several other illnesses came to be classified as AIDS defining illnesses.

According to the CDC, it is estimated that 1,122,900 people in the USA were living with HIV.

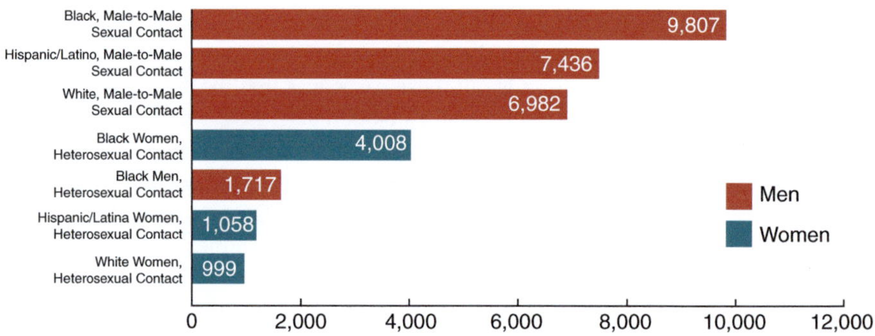

New HIV diagnoses in the US and dependent areas for the most-affected subpopulations, 2017. HIV in the United States and Dependent Areas. (2019, October 30). Retrieved from https://www.cdc.gov/hiv/statistics/overview/ataglance.html

Bottom Line

These five cases of PJP in Los Angeles were the start of the medical and public health communities' awareness of the HIV/AIDS epidemic in the USA. The central distribution of a not yet available treatment for PCP was a crucial piece in the discovery of the AIDS epidemic that was presenting in many cities around the country with many separate manifestations related to acquired immunodeficiencies and opportunistic infections. In 1982 the CDC had reports of PCP in several patients with hemophilia. The virus itself was not discovered until 1983 and the use of AZT (zidovudine) did not emerge until 1987. While there has been much progress in the prevention and treatment of HIV/AIDS since then, it continues to affect a staggering amount of people and its transmission continues to be a public health matter of great concern.

Reference

1. Walzer PD, et al. Pneumocystis carinii pneumonia in the United States. Epidemiologic, diagnostic, and clinical features. Ann Intern Med. 1974;80:83–93.

Chapter 29
Decision for Hospital Admission for Community Acquired Pneumonia (PORT)-1997

Chris Azzolino

Background

There is a great deal of variety in hospitalization rates in patients with community acquired pneumonia. Physicians often rely on a patient's clinical appearance and subjective impressions to help determine need for hospitalization. Accurate and objective models of prognosis would help physician's decision making, particularly in determining that a patient is at low risk of death without the need for hospitalization.

Objective

To develop a prediction rule for patients who are at low risk of death within 30 days of presentation.

Fine, M. J. (1997). A prediction rule to identify low-risk patients with community acquired pneumonia. *The New England Journal Of Medicine*, *336*(4), 243–250.
Hyperlink to PDF: https://www.nejm.org/doi/pdf/10.1056/NEJM199701233360402?articleTools=true

---

C. Azzolino (✉)
Jefferson Health, Abington, PA, USA
e-mail: christopher.azzolino@jefferson.edu

J. Russell, N. S. Skolnik (eds.), *Top Articles in Primary Care*,
https://doi.org/10.1007/978-3-031-25620-2_29

Design and Methods

- The study included just over 14,000 adult inpatients with community acquired pneumonia in a retrospective chart review study.
- Prediction rule was assigned to patients and groups them into 5 risk classes based on score. Rule was derived from PORT cohort study in 1991.
- The rule assigns points based on age and presence of coexisting disease, abnormal physical exam findings, and abnormal lab findings at presentation
- Rule was designed in 2 steps. Step 1 designed to identify a subgroup of patients at low risk of death solely based on history and physical. Step 2 designed to quantify the risk of death in patients with same findings used in step 1 plus laboratory/radiographic data
- Established 30-day hospital mortality as the outcome

Results

- No significant differences in mortality in each of the five risk classes
- Risk class was significantly associated with the risk of subsequent hospitalization among those treated as well as use of intensive care and number of days in the hospital among inpatients
- Only 0.4% of the pneumonia patients in the lowest risk group died (and none in the outpatients in that group).
- Of the lowest risk group of outpatients, only 5.1% required subsequent admission.
- In the highest risk class, 29.2% of the patients died and 17.3% ended up in intensive care with 72% remaining in hospital over 7 days.

Importance

- Demonstrates the very broad prognosis for patients with community acquired pneumonia, ranging from rapid recovery to death, important to be able to differentiate which way a patient will head
- Serves as a tool to help physicians make more rational decisions about hospitalization for patients with pneumonia. Gives objective evidence for clinical decisions.
- Accurately identifies patients with community acquired pneumonia who are at low risk for death and other adverse outcomes
- Served for the groundwork of the "Pneumonia Severity Index" which has been used since as a prediction rule for probability of morbidity and mortality among patients with community acquired pneumonia, specifically for if a patient is to go home, go to medical floor, or go to ICU.

Updates

- CURB-65 developed in 2002 was which served at a better triage tool if a patient should be admitted or to be discharged home. Was deemed to be helpful for the emergency room and much more rapid and quick then the Pneumonia Severity Index. 1 point for each category. >1 = inpatient. 0–1 = consider outpatient.

  C = confusion
  U = uremia (BUN > 20)
  R = respiratory rate > 30
  B = blood pressure < 90
  Age > 65

Bottom Line

- Uses objective evidence based on age, altered mental status, vital signs, past medical history, gender, physical exam findings, and laboratory findings
- This study gives a prediction rule which helps identify patients with community acquired pneumonia who are low risk and gives objective evidence to help aid in clinical decision-making regarding disposition.

Chapter 30
Blood Testing for Diagnosis of Tuberculosis Infections-2006

Anne Sprogell

Background

It is thought that eradication of tuberculosis might be a realistic goal in countries with a low prevalence. In order for that to happen, diagnosis and treatment of patients with latent disease needs to improve, as they can act as a reservoir. When this article was published in 2006, it was estimated that 9–14 million people living in the USA had latent TB. The standard of care at that time for testing for TB was the tuberculin skin test (TST); however, the TST was known to be unreliable. It often provides false negative results in the immunocompromised and high-risk patients. The TST is also unreliable in patients who have been vaccinated with the BCG TB vaccine, often providing false positive results. QuantiFERON-TB Gold and T-SPOT.*TB,* two interferon gamma release assays, were developed to hopefully provide a more accurate test than the TST.

Objective

The goal of this paper was to compare the tuberculin skin test and two blood tests (T-SPOT.*TB* and QuantiFERON-TB Gold) to see if there could be a more reliable test than the TST.

Ferrara, G. et al (2006). Use in routine clinical practice of two commercial blood tests for diagnosis of infection with Mycobacterium tuberculosis: a prospective study. *The Lancet*, *367*(9519), 1328–1334. doi: 10.1016/s0140-6736(06)68579 6

A. Sprogell (✉)
Jefferson Health, Abington, PA, USA

J. Russell, N. S. Skolnik (eds.), *Top Articles in Primary Care*,
https://doi.org/10.1007/978-3-031-25620-2_30

Results

Both blood tests had similar agreement overall with the skin test but showed some improvement over the TST in certain populations. While the skin test can be positive for people with BCG vaccination, both blood tests came back positive for fewer BCG vaccinated test subjects. The QuantiFERON-TB Gold had more indeterminate results than the T-SPOT.*TB*. Patients on immunosuppressive therapy had more indeterminate results for both blood tests. QuantiFERON-TB Gold had more indeterminate results in patients under 5 years of age than T-SPOT.*TB*. The paper concluded that the blood tests are more specific than the skin test. The two blood tests differ in rates of indeterminate and positive results and led the authors to suggest that each blood test might be better in certain clinical situations [1].

Importance

The introduction of QuantiFERON-TB Gold and T-SPOT.*TB* suggested that perhaps there was a better way to test for TB than the TST. Both blood tests were better than the skin test in patients who had been vaccinated with BCG. A one step blood test would be easier for patients and medical staff, as the patient would not have to come back for a second visit and it would remove the inconsistency inherent in the TST, which asked different providers to both place the test and evaluate the results.

Updates

These two blood tests (IGRAs) have become an important part of the standard testing for latent tuberculosis. Below are the guidelines from AAFP [2]:

- In patients who are likely to be infected with a high risk of progression and are older than 5 years of age: both IGRA and the Tuberculin Skin Test (TST) are acceptable, although one should consider dual testing and a positive result on either would be considered positive.
- In patients who are likely to be infected with a high risk of progression and are 5 years old or younger: the TST is preferred, although IGRAs are acceptable and dual testing should be considered, with a positive result on either being considered positive.
- In patients who are likely to be infected with a low to intermediate risk of progression: an IGRA is preferred, but TST is acceptable
- In patients who are unlikely to be infected: testing is not recommended, but if it has to be done, IGRAs are preferred and the TST is acceptable. One can consider repeat or dual testing where a negative result on either would be considered negative.

Bottom Line

IGRAs (interferon gamma release assays) such as T-SPOT.*TB* and QuantiFERON-TB Gold are an acceptable and often preferable test for latent TB in most populations and are often easier for patients and practitioners to utilize. In certain populations, it can be helpful to do dual testing with IGRAs and TST.

References

1. Ferrara G, Losi M, Damico R, Roversi P, Piro R, Meacci M, et al. Use in routine clinical practice of two commercial blood tests for diagnosis of infection with Mycobacterium tuberculosis: a prospective study. Lancet. 2006;367(9519):1328–34. https://doi.org/10.1016/s0140-6736(06)68579-6.
2. Hauk L. Tuberculosis: guidelines for diagnosis from the ATS, IDSA, and CDC. 2018. Retrieved from https://www.aafp.org/afp/2018/0101/p56.html.

Chapter 31
Prophylaxis to Prevent HIV Infections (PREP)-2010

Dat Tran and William Callahan

Background

- Men and transgender women (MtF) who have sex with men are at increased risk of HIV. Protocols have been established for post-exposure chemoprophylaxis for HIV exposure but are hard to consistently provide and can be confusing. This article explores the possibility of Pre-exposure prophylaxis (PrEP) to combat the HIV epidemic that disproportionately affects the gay male community.

Objective

- To determine the safety and efficacy of combination Emtricitabine and Tenofovir (FTC-TDF), two established anti-retrovirals, in reducing the incidence of HIV in men and transgender women who have sex with men.

Grant, R. M. (2010). Preexposure chemoprophylaxis for HIV prevention in men who have sex with men. The New England Journal of Medicine, 363(27), 2587–2599.
Hyperlink to PDF: https://www.nejm.org/doi/pdf/10.1056/NEJMoa1011205?articleTools=true

---

D. Tran (✉) · W. Callahan
Jefferson Health, Abington, PA, USA
e-mail: Dat.tran@jefferson.edu; William.callahan@jefferson.edu

J. Russell, N. S. Skolnik (eds.), *Top Articles in Primary Care*,
https://doi.org/10.1007/978-3-031-25620-2_31

Design and Methods

- 2499 HIV-negative, adult men and transgender women who have sex with men were randomly assigned to be given daily oral combo antiretroviral FTC-TDF or placebo.
- The two groups had similar characteristics such as age, ethnicity, and rates of high-risk sexual behavior, including unprotected sex with men and drug use.
- Participants were seen every 4 weeks where they were tested for HIV, tested and treated for other STDs, provided comprehensive risk-reduction counseling, given condoms, and assessed for adherence with their assigned treatment: daily FTC-TDF or placebo.
- Adherence was determined based on pharmacy dispense data, pill counts, and self-reported data. Subjects were "on treatment" if their calculated pill use was $\geq$50% of days.
- Interval testing for HIV consisted of 2 rapid antibody tests each time. Positive tests were confirmed with a Western blot analysis of serum. Newly diagnosed HIV infections were RNA tested to determine first date of laboratory evidence of infection, tested for resistance to HIV medications, and the individual was treated with the standard of care.
- Drug levels for FTC-TDF were measured in the plasma and peripheral-blood mononuclear cells of HIV-positive subjects and a cohort of HIV-negative subjects in the treatment group.
- Subjects were monitored for adverse drug reactions via self-report and laboratory testing.

Results

- Subjects were followed for a median of 1.2 years.
- 100 subjects were infected with HIV after enrollment, 36 in the FTC-TDF group and 64 in the placebo group, indicating a 44% reduction of incidence of HIV ($P = 0.05$).
- In the treatment arm, only 3 of 34 (9%) HIV-infected subjects had detectable levels of FTC-TDF, compared to 22 of 41 (54%) of seronegative control subjects.
- Of the 3 HIV-positive subjects with detectable drug levels, none was higher than the median for the seronegative control.
- In the treatment arm, there is a 95% relative risk reduction between subjects with a detectable drug level and subjects without a detectable drug level when adjusted for reported unprotected receptive anal intercourse, the main mode of HIV transmission in the study population.
- Common side effects of the FTC-TDF regimen were nausea and creatinine elevation.

Importance

I remember the visit vividly. I had seen the patient for evaluation of lymphadenopathy. A workup revealed only one lab abnormality: the patient had become HIV positive, a new development compared to their last test 2 months prior. What became clear after the fact was that the patient had been in an HIV discordant relationship. The patient had been HIV negative, and their partner had been HIV positive, though the patient only became aware of this discordance shortly before their own diagnosis. It highlighted for me the potential for benefit from PrEP, and the need for uptake by primary care providers.

Pre-Exposure Prophylaxis against HIV represents one of the few times we have seen a major push to prophylactically treat a population with medication for the prevention of viral illness. What began in the 1980s as a major public health scare after the recognition of what at the time was known as Gay-Related Immunodeficiency (GRID) has largely evolved into a chronic illness. However, the emotional, mental, and economic burdens of the diagnosis remain. The recognition today of the ability to prevent its transmission represents a huge milestone in the battling of this illness. The most common forms of PrEP today, both available in oral form, have well-tolerated side effects and any concerning developments tend to resolve after discontinuation.

Currently, PrEP is recommended for those considered highest risk, including men who have sex with men, IV drug users, and those in a sero-discordant relationship. Further, it is now recommended that all sexually active adolescents and adults be educated on PrEP, and if engaging in high-risk sexual activity, be offered to start on PrEP. As with all guidelines, each of these recommendations should be individualized to the patient.

It remains important for primary care providers to be aware of PrEP and be comfortable with its initiation. The future of PrEP appears promising. Only very recently did an injectable form of PrEP become available, though the oral form remains the more popular version at this time. Studies into an implantable form of PrEP look promising, but as of this time none has been approved.

Bottom Line

- Today, HIV is much more treatable, but still carries a large emotional and physiologic toll on the patient, with an economic burden in the form of medical care and lost work.
- HIV disproportionately affects multiple groups, including people of color, men and transgendered women who have sex with men, and IV drug users. Pre-exposure prophylaxis that is safe, effective, and easy to implement represents a milestone in medicine, attempting to prevent this illness before exposure. Medical providers should be aware of PREP and discuss it with their patients.

Chapter 32
URI Prescription Management-2016

Angela Kalinowski

Background

Respiratory diseases are one of the most common reasons for visits with family physicians. Most respiratory infections are self-limiting, and previous systematic reviews have suggested that antibiotics only slightly modify the course of most of these infections. Nevertheless, in the USA, about 60% of patients with a sore throat and 71% of patients with acute uncomplicated bronchitis still receive an antibiotic prescription, overprescription of which increases resistance to these drugs. Overprescription of antibiotics also strains resources, places patients at risk of adverse effects, and increases the number of future appointments for similar complaints. When it is difficult to determine whether an infection is caused by a virus or bacteria, the delayed antibiotic prescribing strategy can be a valuable tool to avoid unnecessary antibiotic use. This approach is described as prescribing an antibiotic to take only if the symptoms worsen or if there is no improvement several days after the medical visit. A previous study in Spain evaluated delayed prescribing in primary care and found a reduction of antibiotic prescribing but did not include clinical

---

Abad, M. D. L. P., Dalmau, G. M., Bakedano, M. M., González, A. I. G., Criado, Y. C., Anadón, S. H., … Alonso-Coello, P. (2016). Prescription Strategies in Acute Uncomplicated Respiratory Infections. *JAMA Internal Medicine*, *176*(1), 21. doi: 10.1001/jamainternmed.2015.7088
https://www.researchgate.net/profile/Ana_Gonzalez_Gonzalez/publication/287808773_Prescription_Strategies_in_Acute_Uncomplicated_Respiratory_Infections_A_Randomized_Clinical_Trial/links/56796c9308ae40c0e27dc0af/Prescription-Strategies-in-Acute-Uncomplicated-Respiratory-Infections-A-Randomized-Clinical-Trial.pdf?origin=publication_detail

---

A. Kalinowski (✉)
Jefferson Health, Abington, PA, USA

J. Russell, N. S. Skolnik (eds.), *Top Articles in Primary Care*,
https://doi.org/10.1007/978-3-031-25620-2_32

outcomes. Therefore, this study was designed to determine the effectiveness of two delayed antibiotic strategies compared with immediate antibiotic prescription or no antibiotics.

Objective

To determine the efficacy and safety of two delayed antibiotic strategies in acute, uncomplicated respiratory infections.

Design and Methods

- This study was a pragmatic, randomized, multicenter, clinical trial.
- Eligible patients were older than 18 years and had acute pharyngitis, rhinosinusitis, acute bronchitis, or exacerbation of mild-to-moderate chronic obstructive pulmonary disease.
- Patients were randomized to 1 of 4 strategies:
  - Delayed patient-led prescription strategy where patients were given an antibiotic prescription at the initial visit and given the following instructions on when to consider taking it.
  - Delayed prescription collection strategy requiring patients to collect their prescription from the primary care center reception desk 3 days after initial visit.
  - Immediate prescription strategy where patients received an antibiotic at first visit and were instructed to start the medication on the same day.
  - No antibiotic strategy.
- Delayed prescription strategies consisted of prescribing an antibiotic to take only if the symptoms worsen or if there is no improvement several days after the medical visit.
- Patients allocated to the delayed antibiotic strategies received the same instructions from the physician. They were told it was normal to feel worse over the first few days after the visit. If they felt substantially worse in the first few days, however, they were recommended to consider taking the antibiotics or to return to the physician if they considered it necessary. If they noted no improvement after 5 days (in cases of pharyngitis) or after 10 days (in cases of other infections), they were also instructed to consider taking the antibiotics.
- Patients allocated to the immediate prescription strategy or to the no prescription strategy were told it was normal to feel worse over the first few days after the visit. However, they were instructed to consider consultation again if they felt they should see their physician or if there was no improvement after 5 days (in cases of pharyngitis) or after 10 days (in cases of other infections).
- The choice of antibiotic was made by the physician.

- The primary outcome measure was the duration and severity of symptoms.
- Patients filled out a daily questionnaire for a maximum of 30 days.
- Secondary outcomes were antibiotic use, satisfaction with health care, belief in the effectiveness of antibiotics, and absenteeism (absence from work or doing their daily activities). The risk of complications (e.g., pneumonia, abscesses, or cellulitis) and the need for unscheduled health care were also tracked.
- A central telephone follow-up was conducted on days 2, 7, 15, and 22 if symptoms persisted.

Results

- 398 patients were included in the analysis.
- The mean (SD) duration of severe symptoms was 3.6 (3.3) days for the immediate prescription group and 4.7 (3.6) days for the no prescription group. The median (IQR) duration of severe symptoms was 3 (1–4) days for the prescription collection group and 3 (2–6) days for the patient-led prescription group.
- Patients randomized to the immediate prescription strategy showed shorter durations of severe symptoms, ranging from 0.4 days less than the prescription collection strategy to 1.5 days less than the patient-led prescription strategy. The duration of moderate symptoms was mean (SD) 4.7 (4.0) days for the immediate prescription group; 5.2 (4.3) days for the prescription collection group; 6.0 (5.5) days for the patient-led prescription group; and 6.5 (5.2) days for the no prescription group. The duration of moderate symptoms was significantly shorter for the prescription collection group than for the no prescription group.
- The duration of common symptoms (i.e., fever, discomfort, cough, difficulty sleeping, and difficulty performing daily activities) in the immediate prescription group compared with the no prescription group was shorter for 3 out of 5 symptoms.
- Compared with the no prescription group, the duration of 2 common symptoms was shorter for the patient-led prescription group and shorter for 1 symptom in the prescription collection group.
- In the immediate prescription group, 92 patients (91.1%) used antibiotics, compared with 12 patients (12.1%) in the no prescription group, 23 patients (23.0%) in the prescription collection group, and 32 patients (32.6%) in the patient-led prescription group.
- No differences were observed for complications, adverse effects, or the need for unscheduled care among the strategy groups, and no differences were observed in the perception of general health statuses assessed at 30 days.
- Rates of absenteeism were lower in the delayed strategy groups.
- Belief that antibiotics had no effect or were not very effective was higher for patients in the 2 delayed antibiotic strategies and the no antibiotic strategy.
- More patients randomized to the immediate prescription strategy reported that they would return to their physician for a similar episode than patients in the other strategies.

Importance

It was found in this study that the delayed strategy groups had slightly greater symptom burden and duration than the immediate prescription group, although the differences were not clinically relevant. Delayed prescription and no prescription strategies notably reduced antibiotic use compared with the immediate prescription group. A delayed antibiotic strategy may be helpful compared with a no prescription strategy when patients or physicians are concerned about the risk of complications, or when patients expect to be prescribed antibiotics, in order to attempt to reduce overprescription of antibiotics.

Bottom Line

In order to address overprescription of antibiotics for usually self-limited infections of the respiratory system, a study was conducted comparing four antibiotic prescribing strategies: delayed patient-led prescription, delayed prescription collection strategy, immediate prescription, and no antibiotic prescription. It was shown that the delayed strategy groups had slightly greater symptom burden and duration than the immediate prescription group, although the differences were not clinically relevant. Delayed prescription and no prescription strategies notably reduced antibiotic use compared with the immediate prescription group. These strategies can be employed to attempt to decrease overprescription of antibiotics in order to reduce antibiotic resistant and adverse effects from antibiotics.

Part VI
Lipids

John Russell

Chapter 33
Lipid Lowering in Coronary Artery Disease (4S)-1994

Anupriya Grover-Wenk

Background

Before the 4S trial, drug therapy for hypercholesterolemia had been controversial because there was insufficient data to prove that any form of drug therapy improved survival in patients with known coronary heart disease (CHD). At the time that the 4S study group was formed, the Expert's Panel in Europe and the USA had started recommending that lowering cholesterol, specifically low-density lipoprotein C (LDL-C), through dietary changes, and that possible use of cholesterol lowering agents could be beneficial in prolonging life in patients with CHD. The 4S trial was the first to show that treatment of hypercholesterolemia with a statin resulted in a decreased mortality rate of 30% and cardiovascular events in a high-risk secondary prevention population.

Objective

- To investigate whether the cholesterol-lowering agent, Simvastatin, has an effect on morbidity and mortality in patients with a history of previous myocardial infarction (MI) or angina, who also had moderately raised cholesterol, between 5.5 and 8.0 mmol/L (212–309 mg/dL).

Scandinavian Simvastatin Survival Study Group, (1994). Lancet (London, England), 344(8934), 1383–1389.
Hyperlink to PDF: https://www.thelancet.com/pb/assets/raw/Lancet/pdfs/issue-10000/4s-statins.pdf

A. Grover-Wenk (✉)
Jefferson Health, Abington, PA, USA
e-mail: Anupriya.Grover@jefferson.edu

J. Russell, N. S. Skolnik (eds.), *Top Articles in Primary Care*,
https://doi.org/10.1007/978-3-031-25620-2_33

- A second objective was to investigate whether the incidence of major coronary events (fatal and non-fatal MI and sudden death) could be reduced with Simvastatin.

Design and Methods

- The 4S study was a multi-center, randomized, double blind, placebo controlled clinical trial which recruited 4444 patients from 7027 patients who had been following dietary recommendations for 2 months.
- All participants were at high risk for death given their history of CHD and were selected from 94 clinical centers in Denmark, Finland, Norway, and Sweden from 1988 to 1989 and were aged between 35 and 70 years old, with an average age of 59.
- Patients were only recruited if they met all exclusion criteria and had a baseline fasting serum cholesterol >5.5 mmol/L; these patients were then given dietary advice to follow for 8 weeks.
- If after 8 weeks, serum cholesterol was 5.5–8.0 mmol/L and triglycerides were ≤2.5 mmol/L, the patient was randomly assigned to treatment with Simvastatin 20 mg or placebo.
- The Simvastatin dose was adjusted, if necessary, at the 12-week and 6-month visits based on serum total cholesterol; the goal was to reduce total serum cholesterol to 3.0–5.2 mmol/L.
- Of the 4444 total subjects enrolled, 3617 were men and 827 were women; 2223 were assigned to a placebo and 2221 were given 20–40 mg of Simvastatin daily.
- The study continued for a median period of 5.4 years, and the patients in the treatment group were followed for an additional 5 years.

Results

- After 5.4 years, the patients taking Simvastatin showed a 35% reduction in LDL-C and a 30% reduction in overall mortality.
- The risk of non-fatal MI reduced by 37% and fatal and non-fatal cerebrovascular events, such as stroke and TIA, decreased by 28%.
- The number needed to treat was 30.
- Lipid concentrations seen in the placebo group did not change dramatically; however, there was an upward trend in serum triglycerides.
- Despite the study only having 827 (19%) women, it was shown that Simvastatin did reduce the risk of major coronary events (34%) to about the same extent of men in the treatment group.
- The small number of women in the study, as well as the small number of deaths of women in the study, prevented an accurate assessment of Simvastatin on all-cause mortality or CHD mortality in women.

- A subgroup analysis of patients with diabetes in the 4S trial showed a 55% reduction for major CHD events; the reduction in total mortality for this subgroup was 29%.
- The 4S trial was the first study to show that cholesterol-lowering therapy in CHD patients ≥65 years of age reduced the risk of all-cause mortality and major coronary events; Simvastatin treatment showed a 34% reduction in risk for all-cause mortality which was attributed to 43% reduction in risk for CHD mortality in this subgroup.
- Simvastatin therapy was generally well tolerated and only 6% of patients in both groups discontinued the study drug due to adverse events; a single case of rhabdomyolysis occurred in a woman taking Simvastatin 20 mg daily and recovered when she discontinued treatment.

Importance

Before the 4S trial, Britain had been embroiled in a controversy over the role of cholesterol in CHD. It was believed that cholesterol played a causal role in atherosclerosis and cardiovascular disease. This theory was known as "the lipid hypothesis". It took until the 4S trial to prove this relationship and expand upon it.

The 4S trial was a multi-center, randomized, double blind, placebo controlled clinical trial, and the first of its kind to show that treatment of a secondary prevention population with a statin decreased mortality and cardiovascular events by 30% in patients with a history of MI or angina pectoris. While the results were underpowered, the study results also had secondary effects and showed its benefit in women, patients with diabetes, and those ≥65 years of age. Most patients tolerated simvastatin well and few adverse side effects were reported. In addition, long-term follow-up of the 4S treatment arm patients showed no increase in rates of cancer with the long-term use of simvastatin. The long-term effects seen over 10 years resulted in a 17% reduction in cardiovascular mortality and a 24% reduction in coronary related deaths in the 2221 patients who continued simvastatin. Before this study was published, many researchers believed that statins could cause cancer. However, the data in the 4S trial showed that long-term statin users actually have a slightly reduced cancer risk, but this finding was not statistically significant.

Updates

- The study subjects receiving simvastatin were followed for 5 years in a post-trial follow-up to examine the effects of cholesterol lowering treatment on mortality and risk of cancer.

  - The findings were consistent with the first part of the study and showed continued survival benefits while also showing no increased risk of developing cancer.
  - While it was noted that there were fewer cancer-related deaths in those study subjects on simvastatin, these results were not statistically significant.

- The results of the 4S trial have been replicated many times and in a meta-analysis of 10 trials since 2002, statins were shown to reduce coronary events, stroke, and all-cause mortality without increasing non-coronary mortality.
  - Only in 4 out of 5 trials using pravastatin, an increase of cancer was noted in the pravastatin arm (5%); however, this was not found to be statistically significant; pravastatin was also found to be less effective in preventing stroke than other statins.
  - Long-term studies are needed to understand the long-term effects of statins on cancer, as it has been found to be carcinogenic in certain animal models
  - Many of the statin trials have had low number of women participants and in the studies that did include women, it was shown that female patients benefit equally in the use of Simvastatin as male patients.

Bottom Line

- The 4S trial shows that lipid lowering agents such as simvastatin decreased mortality and coronary related events in patients with CHD. In addition, this finding persisted over the course of following the treatment group for a total of 10 years, and further, showed that there was no increased incidence of developing cancer while on simvastatin for a prolonged period.

Chapter 34
Intensive Versus Moderate Lipid Lowering for Acute Coronary Syndrome-2004

Evan R. Gooberman

Background

Heart disease is the leading cause of death in the USA [1]. Higher cholesterol levels increase the risk of coronary heart disease [2]. Cholesterol-lowering therapy with 3-hydroxy-3-methylglutaryl coenzyme A reductase inhibitors (statins) has been shown to reduce the risk of death and cardiovascular events [3].

Objective

- Assess the optimal level of low-density lipoprotein (LDL) cholesterol levels—specifically to assess if there is a benefit to using high-intensity statin over moderate-intensity statin.

Cannon CP, Braunwald E, et al. Intensive versus Moderate Lipid Lowering with Statins after Acute Coronary Syndromes. N Engl J Med 2004; 350:1595–1504.
Hyperlink to article: https://www.nejm.org/doi/pdf/10.1056/NEJMoa040583?articleTools=true

E. R. Gooberman (✉)
Jefferson Health, Abington, PA, USA

J. Russell, N. S. Skolnik (eds.), *Top Articles in Primary Care*,
https://doi.org/10.1007/978-3-031-25620-2_34

Design and Methods

- Four thousand one hundred sixty-two patients who had been hospitalized for an acute coronary syndrome within the previous 10 days and had a total cholesterol equal to or less than 240 mg/dL were randomized in a double-blind, double-dummy study.
- Primary endpoints: death from any cause, myocardial infarction, documented unstable angina requiring rehospitalization, revascularization, and stroke.
- Patients received standard medical and interventional treatment for acute coronary syndrome in addition to being assigned to one of the two groups: 40 mg pravastatin daily (moderate-intensity statin) or 80 mg atorvastatin daily (high-intensity statin).
- Patients were followed for 18–36 months (24 month average) until 925 events had been reported, at which point all participants returned for a final study visit—8 patients (0.2%) were lost to follow-up.
- Data was preliminarily evaluated with an intention-to-treat analysis, with a transition to two-sided confidence intervals.

Results

- The median LDL cholesterol level in the moderate-intensity pravastatin group was 95 mg/dL, and the median LDL cholesterol level in the high-intensity atorvastatin group was 62 mg/dL ($p < 0.001$).
- Using the high-intensity atorvastatin resulted in a 16% risk reduction in the hazard ratio for the studied end points compared to the moderate-intensity pravastatin—there was a 25% risk reduction when looking at the risk of death, myocardial infarction, and urgent revascularization.
- The benefits of using the high-intensity atorvastatin compared to the moderate-intensity pravastatin were noticeable as early as 30 days and were consistent throughout the study.

Importance

It has been common practice to prescribe statins to lower cholesterol and reduce the risk of acute coronary syndrome, but until the PROVE IT study, it was unclear if the intensity of the statin was contributory. Now there is evidence to support prescribing higher intensity statins to lower the LDL cholesterol levels more than moderate-intensity statins and improve morbidity and mortality.

Bottom Line

- Intensive therapy with high-dose atorvastatin resulted in a lower LDL level than standard-dose pravastatin, and this was associated with a statistically significant clinical benefit.
- High-dose statins are the standard or care for secondary prevention in coronary artery disease and cerebrovascular disease and high risk states like diabetes and peripheral vascular diseases.

References

1. Murphy SL, Xu JQ, Kochanek KD, Arias E. Mortality in the United States, 2017. NCHS Data Brief, no 328. Hyattsville: National Center for Health Statistics; 2018.
2. Dawber TR, Moore FE, Mann GV. Coronary heart disease in the Framingham study. Am J Public Health. 1957;47:4–24.
3. Heart Protection Study Collaborative Group. MRC/BHF Heart Protection Study of cholesterol lowering with simvastatin in 20,536 high-risk individuals: a randomized placebo-controlled trial. Lancet. 2002;360:7–22.

Chapter 35
Preventing Vascular Events with Rosuvastatin in Patients with Elevated CRP (JUPITER)-2008

Angela Kalinowski

Background

Statin therapy is recommended for the prevention of myocardial infarction, stroke, and death from cardiovascular causes for patients with established vascular disease, diabetes, and overt hyperlipidemia. However, half of all myocardial infarctions and strokes occur among apparently healthy men and women with levels of low-density lipoprotein (LDL) cholesterol that are below currently recommended thresholds for treatment. Elevated levels of the inflammatory biomarker high-sensitivity C-reactive protein have been previously shown to predict cardiovascular events. Statin therapy has previously been shown to reduce levels of high-sensitivity C-reactive protein. However, no trial has directly addressed the question of whether persons with LDL cholesterol levels below current treatment thresholds but with elevated high-sensitivity C-reactive protein level might benefit from statin therapy from a cardiovascular standpoint.

Ridker, P. M., Danielson, E., Fonseca, F. A., Genest, J., Gotto, A. M., Kastelein, J. J., … Glynn, R. J. (2008). Rosuvastatin to Prevent Vascular Events in Men and Women with Elevated C-Reactive Protein. New England Journal of Medicine, 359(21), 2195–2207. doi: 10.1056/nejmoa0807646. https://www.nejm.org/doi/pdf/10.1056/NEJMoa0807646?articleTools=true

---

A. Kalinowski (✉)
Jefferson Health, Abington, PA, USA

J. Russell, N. S. Skolnik (eds.), *Top Articles in Primary Care*,
https://doi.org/10.1007/978-3-031-25620-2_35

Objective

- The primary objective of the Justification for the Use of Statins in Prevention: an Intervention Trial Evaluating Rosuvastatin (JUPITER) was to investigate whether treatment with rosuvastatin, 20 mg daily, as compared with placebo, would decrease the rate of first major cardiovascular events.

Design and Methods

- This study was a randomized, double-blind, placebo controlled, multicenter trial conducted at 1315 sites in 26 countries.
- Men 50 years of age or older and women 60 years of age or older who did not have a history of cardiovascular disease and had an LDL cholesterol level of less than 130 mg/dL and a high-sensitivity C-reactive protein level of 2.0 mg/L or more were eligible for the trial.
- Participants were also required to have a triglyceride level of less than 500 mg/dL.
- Exclusion criteria were previous or current use of lipid-lowering therapy, current use of postmenopausal hormone-replacement therapy, evidence of hepatic dysfunction, a creatine kinase level that was more than three times the upper limit of the normal range, a creatinine level that was higher than 2.0 mg/dL, diabetes, uncontrolled hypertension, cancer within 5 years before enrollment, uncontrolled hypothyroidism, and a recent history of alcohol or drug abuse or another medical condition that might compromise safety or the successful completion of the study.
- Patients with inflammatory conditions such as severe arthritis, lupus, or inflammatory bowel disease were excluded, as were patients taking immunosuppressant agents.
- Eligible subjects were randomly assigned to receive either rosuvastatin, 20 mg daily, or placebo.
- Follow-up visits were scheduled to occur at 13 weeks and 6, 12, 18, 24, 30, 36, 42, 48, 54, and 60 months after randomization.
- Follow-up assessments included laboratory evaluations, pill counts, and structured interviews assessing outcomes and potential adverse events.
- Measurements of lipid levels, high-sensitivity C-reactive protein levels, hepatic and renal function, blood glucose levels, and glycated hemoglobin values were performed in a central laboratory.
- The primary outcome was the occurrence of a first major cardiovascular event-nonfatal myocardial infarction, nonfatal stroke, hospitalization for unstable angina, an arterial revascularization procedure, or confirmed death from cardiovascular causes.

Results

- A total of 17,802 people were randomly assigned to participate in the study.
- At baseline, the median LDL cholesterol level was 108 mg/dL, the high-density lipoprotein (HDL) cholesterol level was 49 mg/dL, and the triglyceride level was 118 mg/dL in both groups.
- At baseline, the high-sensitivity C-reactive protein level was 4.2 mg/L in the rosuvastatin group and 4.3 mg/L in the placebo group.
- At the 12-month visit, the rosuvastatin group had a 50% lower median LDL cholesterol level, a 37% lower median high-sensitivity C-reactive protein level, and a 17% lower median triglyceride level compared to the placebo group.
- At the time of study termination 142 first major cardiovascular events had occurred in the rosuvastatin group and 251 in the placebo group.
- Total numbers of reported serious adverse events were similar in the rosuvastatin and placebo groups.
- There were no significant differences between the two study groups with regard to muscle weakness, newly diagnosed cancer, or disorders of the hematologic, gastrointestinal, hepatic, or renal systems.
- Physician-reported diabetes was more frequent in the rosuvastatin group.

Importance

In this randomized trial of apparently healthy men and women with elevated levels of high-sensitivity C-reactive protein, rosuvastatin significantly reduced the incidence of major cardiovascular events, despite the fact that nearly all study participants had lipid levels at baseline that were well below the threshold for treatment according to current prevention guidelines.

Updates

A study published in the Lancet in 2012 titled *Cardiovascular Benefits and Diabetes Risks of Statin Therapy in Primary Prevention: an analysis from the JUPITER trial* reported that the risk of developing diabetes on statin therapy appears limited to those with baseline evidence of impaired fasting glucose, metabolic syndrome, severe obesity, or elevated HbA1c, a group of patients already at high risk for developing diabetes. Within the JUPITER trial, the cardiovascular and mortality benefits of statin therapy exceeded the diabetes hazard in the trial population as a whole, as well as, among those at higher risk for developing diabetes [1].

Bottom Line

The primary objective of the Justification for the Use of Statins in Prevention: an Intervention Trial Evaluating Rosuvastatin (JUPITER) was to investigate whether treatment with rosuvastatin, 20 mg daily, as compared with placebo, would decrease the rate of first major cardiovascular events. This study proved that rosuvastatin significantly reduced the incidence of major cardiovascular events in patients with LDL levels below treatment guidelines and elevated C-reactive protein. There was data that supported an increased incidence of diabetes; however, in further analysis of the data the cardiovascular and mortality benefits of statin therapy exceeded the diabetes hazard in the trial population as a whole as well as among those at higher risk for developing diabetes.

Reference

1. Ridker PM, Pradhan A, Macfadyen JG, Libby P, Glynn RJ. Cardiovascular benefits and diabetes risks of statin therapy in primary prevention: an analysis from the JUPITER trial. Lancet. 2012;380(9841):565–71. https://doi.org/10.1016/s0140-6736(12)61190-8.

Chapter 36
Adding Niacin to Statin Therapy in CAD (AIM-HIGH)-2011

Thomas McGinley

Background

There are over 18 million patients in North America with coronary heart disease (CHD). The target of their management has been through the use of statins to lower low-density lipoprotein (LDL). There is a cohort of these patients that have a mixed dyslipidemia with an elevated triglyceride and low high-density lipoprotein (HDL) level. We know that patients with CHD have residual risk of developing acute coronary syndrome even after reaching their LDL target. The question is whether adding additional medication to the statin therapy can lower the residual risk. Niacin has been used for lipid management since the 1950s. It is the lipid lowering medication with the greatest impact on raising HDL levels [1].

Objective

To investigate whether adding extended release niacin to optimized statin therapy with simvastatin can lower the risk of death for CHD, nonfatal myocardial infarction, ischemic stroke, hospitalization for acute coronary syndrome (ACS), or symptom driven coronary or cerebral revascularization.

The AIM-HIGH investigators. Dec 15, 2011. N Engl J Med 2011; 365:2255–2267. https://www.nejm.org/doi/pdf/10.1056/NEJMoa1107579?articleTools=true

T. McGinley (✉)
St. Luke's Health, Coaldale, PA, USA
e-mail: Thomas.McGinley@sluhn.org

J. Russell, N. S. Skolnik (eds.), *Top Articles in Primary Care*,
https://doi.org/10.1007/978-3-031-25620-2_36

Design and Methods

- There were 3414 patients who had their LDL lowered to 40–80 mg/dL with the use of simvastatin and ezetimibe (if needed) to achieve the desired LDL. The subjects were randomized in a double-blind, placebo-controlled method to receive either placebo or escalating doses of extended release niacin. They were studied for 2 years with a 36 month follow up period.

Results

- After 2 years there was an increase of HDL from 35 to 42 mg/dL and triglycerides lowered from 164 to 122 mg/dL. LDL was also lowered from 74 to 62 mg/dL.
- There was no difference seen in the primary end point with 16.4% in the niacin and 16.2% in the placebo group with a hazard ratio of 1.02.

Importance

This study showed that despite improvements in HDL, triglycerides and LDL that the addition of extended release niacin to a patient optimized on statin therapy made no difference on cardiovascular outcomes.

Updates

- The study was one in a series of studies that showed underwhelming results from the addition of an additional cholesterol-lowering agents to statin therapy. This included fenofibrate, fish oil, and even ezetimibe, that was part of this study [2–4].
- Icosapent ethyl was released in January of 2020 and has some early promising results on its ability to reduce residual risk in patients with CHD on a statin therapy with elevated triglycerides [5].

Bottom Line

- Niacin, for all its potential promise, with its ability to effect so many aspects of the lipid profile does not reduce the risks of cardiovascular events in patient on optimized statin therapy.

References

1. Med Lett Drugs Ther. 2019;61(1565):17–24.
2. The ACCORD Study Group, et al. Effects of combination lipid therapy in type 2 diabetes mellitus. N Engl J Med. 2010;362:1563.
3. Risk and Prevention Study Collaborative Group, Roncaglioni MC, Tombesi M, et al. n-3 fatty acids in patients with multiple cardiovascular risk factors. N Engl J Med. 2013;368(19):1800–8.
4. Cannon CP, et al. Ezetimibe added to statin therapy after acute coronary syndromes. N Engl J Med. 2015;372:2387.
5. Bhatt DL, Steg PG, Miller M, et al., REDUCE-IT Investigators. Cardiovascular risk reduction with Icosapent ethyl for hypertriglyceridemia. N Engl J Med. 2019;380(1):11–22.

Chapter 37
Novel Non Statin Therapy for Hyperlipidemia-PCSK9-2018

Katherine Fradeneck, Merna Mikhail, and Robert Danoff

Background

Prior to the ODYSSEY OUTCOMES trial, there were many evidence-based treatments available for lowering cholesterol levels to improve cardiovascular event risk. The use of statin therapy to lower cardiovascular risk revolutionized therapy. More current research found that sequence variations in proprotein convertase subtilisin-kexin type 9 (PCSK9) lower low density lipoprotein (LDL) and protect against CHD [1]. The ODYSSEY OUTCOMES trial studied the effect of PCSK9 human monoclonal antibody alirocumab on cardiovascular outcomes after acute coronary syndrome in patients receiving high-intensity statin therapy. It was found that the risk of recurrent ischemic cardiovascular events was lower among those who were treated with alirocumab than the placebo by lowering LDL cholesterol.

Objective

- Does alirocumab improve cardiovascular outcomes after an acute coronary syndrome (ACS) in patients receiving high-intensity statin therapy or the patient's maximum tolerated statin dose.

Gregory G. Schwartz, M.D., Ph.D, P, Gabriel Steg, M.D., Micahel Szarek, Ph.D., Deepak L, Bhatt, M.D., M.P.H., et al. Hyperlink to PDF: https://www.nejm.org/doi/full/10.1056/nejmoa1801174

K. Fradeneck · M. Mikhail · R. Danoff (✉)
Jefferson Health Northeast, Philadelphia, PA, USA
e-mail: Katherine.Fradeneck@jefferson.edu; Merna.Mikhail@jefferson.edu; Robert.danoff@jefferson.edu

J. Russell, N. S. Skolnik (eds.), *Top Articles in Primary Care*,
https://doi.org/10.1007/978-3-031-25620-2_37

Design and Methods

- The ODYSSEY OUTCOMES trial was a multi-center, randomized, double-blind, placebo controlled trial which recruited 18,924 patients 40 years of age or older who had an acute coronary syndrome 1–12 months earlier, had an LDL cholesterol level of at least 70 mg/dL, a non-high density lipoprotein cholesterol level of at least 100 mg/dL, or an apolipoprotein B level of at least 80 mg/dL, and were receiving high-intensity dose statin or the maximum tolerated dose statin [2].
- Lipid levels were measured after at least 2 weeks of treatment with atorvastatin 40–80 mg daily, rosuvastatin 20–40 mg daily, or maximum tolerated dose.
- Patients were administered alirocumab 75 mg or matching placebo by subcutaneous injection every 2 weeks.
- Blinded protocol specific dose-adjustment algorithms were used in the alirocumab group to target an LDL cholesterol level of 25–50 mg/dL and to avoid sustained levels below 15 mg/dL, including substitution placebo for alirocumab for sustained LDL cholesterol levels below 15 mg/dL [3].
- The 18,924 patients were randomized to 1315 sites in 57 countries [4].
- Nine thousand four hundred sixty-two received alirocumab subcutaneous injection every 2 weeks and 9462 were assigned to the placebo group [4].
- The study had median length of follow-up of 2.8 years.

Results

- Mean LDL cholesterol levels in the placebo group at 4 months, 12 months, and 48 months were 93, 96, and 103 mg/dL; mean LDL cholesterol levels in the on-treatment alirocumab group at 4 months, 12 months, and 48 months were 38, 42, and 53 mg/dL [5].
- The alirocumab group had LDL cholesterol levels that were an average of 62.7%, 61.0%, and 54.7% lower than the placebo group [5].
- The primary end points (composite of death from coronary heart disease, nonfatal myocardial infarction, fatal or nonfatal ischemic stroke, or unstable angina requiring hospitalization) occurred in 9.5% of patients in the alirocumab group, 11.1% in the placebo group [5].
- The number needed to treat is 49 patients for 4 years to prevent occurrence of one primary end point event [5].
- The incidence of composite primary end points in the placebo group was greatest in patients with LDL cholesterol levels ≥100 mg/dL.
- The greatest absolute reduction in risk with alirocumab was seen in patients with a baseline LDL cholesterol of ≥100 mg/dL.
- The number needed to treat is 16 patients for 4 years to prevent one primary end point in patients with a baseline LDL cholesterol of ≥100 mg/dL [6].
- Alirocumab therapy overall was well tolerated except for mild self-limiting injection-site reactions occurring in 3.8% of the alirocumab group vs. 2.1% in the placebo group [7].

Importance

To this day, cardiac disease remains one of the leading causes of mortality in the developed world. In the effort to reduce the burden of these events on individuals and the healthcare system, more advanced and preventative measures need to be considered. Prior to the ODYSSEY OUTCOMES trial, there were no studies that evaluated the effect of PCSK9 inhibition in conjunction with high intensity or highest tolerated statin in individuals who had established ACS.

The ODYSSEY OUTCOMES was a multi-center, randomized, double-blind, placebo-controlled trial. It showed that the risk of having another major adverse cardiovascular event in patients with ACS decreased by 15% relative to the placebo group; this was implemented with a blinded dose-adjustment strategy to achieve a target range of LDL-C, a known risk factor contributing to cardiac disease.

There are two prior trials that studied the effects of PCSK9 inhibitors, FOURIER (evolocumab) and SPIRE (bococizumab). All these studies did enforce that the overall reduction of LDL using PCSK9 inhibitors did reduce major adverse cardiovascular events in patients with high LDL levels. However, ODYSSEY OUTCOMES was the first to have a longer duration of follow-up, which has facilitated the evaluation of safety.

Updates

While there have been no further studies to verify the effectiveness of PCSK9 inhibitors reducing cardiac event in individuals with known ACS, the EVOPACS trial did study inpatient addition of PCSK9 inhibitors to high-intensity statin therapy in patients hospitalized for ACS [8].

- Three hundred and eight patients hospitalized for ACS with elevated LDL-C levels qualified for this study. Criteria for elevated LDL-C included ≥70 mg/dL on high-intensity statin for at least 4 weeks; ≥90 mg/dL on low- or moderate-intensity statin; or ≥125 mg/dL on no statin. Patients were randomly assigned to receive evolocumab or placebo, as well as atorvastatin 40 mg. LDL-C levels were assessed after 8 weeks. 95.7% of patients in the evolocumab group were found to be at goal vs. 37.6% in the placebo group.
- This study showed that PCSK9 inhibitors are also safe in acute ACS events as adverse events were similar in both groups.
- In addition, while clinical cardiovascular endpoints were not evaluated, intensive reduction of LDL-C level is likely to be efficient in reducing cardiovascular events in patients with the highest risk of those events [9].

Bottom Line

- The ODYSSEY OUTCOMES trial showed that human monoclonal antibody to PCSK9, alirocumab, lowered the risk of major adverse cardiovascular events in patients with previous ACS and whose LDL cholesterol levels remained high despite high-intensity statin therapy or maximum tolerated dose of statin therapy [10].

References

1. Cohen JC, Boerwinkle E, Mosley TH Jr, Hobbs HH. Sequence variations in *PCSK9*, low LDL, and protection against coronary heart disease. N Engl J Med. 2006;354:1264–72.
2. Schwartz GG, Steg PG, Szarek M, et al. Alirocumab and cardiovascular outcomes after acute coronary syndrome. N Engl J Med. 2018;379(22):2097–107, 7–10.
3. Schwartz GG, Steg PG, Szarek M, et al. Alirocumab and cardiovascular outcomes after acute coronary syndrome. N Engl J Med. 2018;379(22):2097–107, 90–6.
4. Schwartz GG, Steg PG, Szarek M, et al. Alirocumab and cardiovascular outcomes after acute coronary syndrome. N Engl J Med. 2018;379(22):2097–107, 148–9.
5. Schwartz GG, Steg PG, Szarek M, et al. Alirocumab and cardiovascular outcomes after acute coronary syndrome. N Engl J Med. 2018;379(22):2097–107, 183–92.
6. Schwartz GG, Steg PG, Szarek M, et al. Alirocumab and cardiovascular outcomes after acute coronary syndrome. N Engl J Med. 2018;379(22):2097–107, 202–3.
7. Schwartz GG, Steg PG, Szarek M, et al. Alirocumab and cardiovascular outcomes after acute coronary syndrome. N Engl J Med. 2018;379(22):2097–107, 214–5.
8. Koskinas KC, Windecker S, Pedrazzini G, et al. Evolocumab for early reduction of LDL cholesterol levels in patients with acute coronary syndromes (EVOPACS). J Am Coll Cardiol. 2019;74(20):2452–62.
9. Silverman MG, Ference BA, Kyungah IM, et al. Association between lowering LDL-C and cardiovascular risk reduction among different therapeutic interventions. JAMA. 2016;316(12):1289–97.
10. Schwartz GG, Steg PG, Szarek M, et al. Alirocumab and cardiovascular outcomes after acute coronary syndrome. N Engl J Med. 2018;379(22):2097–107, 28–30.

Chapter 38
Icosapent Ethyl for Elevated Triglycerides2019

Diana Bonaccorsi and Danielle Carcia

Background

Elevated triglyceride levels are an independent risk factor for ischemic cardiac events. Prior to the REDUCE-IT trial, studies of the treatment of hypertriglyceridemia were not shown to prevent cardiovascular events [1].

Icosapent ethyl is a high-dose marine omega-3 fatty acid. Icosapent ethyl is suspected to have significant anti-inflammatory effects in addition to effectively lowering triglycerides. The REDUCE-IT trial was designed to test if icosapent ethyl, unlike previous treatments for hypertriglyceridemia, would reduce ischemic cardiovascular events.

Objective

- To identify whether icosapent ethyl decreases ischemic cardiac events as defined as cardiovascular death, nonfatal myocardial infarction, nonfatal stroke, coronary revascularization, and unstable angina.

Deepak L. Bhatt, MD., MPH., P. Gabriel Steg, M.D., Michael Miller, M.D., Eliot A. Brinton, M.D., Terry A. Jacobson, MD., Steven B. Ketchum, Ph.D., Ralph T. Doyle, Jr., B.A., Rebecca A. Juliano, PhD., Lixia Jiao, Ph.D., Craig Granowitz, M.D., Ph.D., Jean-Claude Tardif, M.D., and Christie M. Ballantyne, M.D., for the REDUCE-IT Investigators.
Article PDF: https://www.nejm.org/doi/full/10.1056/nejmoa1812792

D. Bonaccorsi · D. Carcia (✉)
Capital Health, Trenton, NJ, USA
e-mail: DCarcia@capitalhealth.org

J. Russell, N. S. Skolnik (eds.), *Top Articles in Primary Care*,
https://doi.org/10.1007/978-3-031-25620-2_38

Design and Methods

- Phase 3b randomized, double-blind, placebo-controlled trial.
- Icosapent ethyl dose 2 g twice daily with food for a total daily dose of 4 g vs. placebo.
- Four hundred seventy-three sites; 11 countries, 19,212 patients screened with 8179 accepted into the study.
- Eligibility Criteria:
  - Forty-five years or older with established cardiovascular disease (secondary prevention cohort)
  - Fifty years or older with diabetes mellitus and one additional risk factor (primary prevention cohort)
  - Fasting triglyceride level of 150–499 mg/dL and LDL between 41 and 100 mg/dL on a stable statin dose for at least 4 weeks
- Primary endpoint was a composite of cardiovascular death, nonfatal myocardial infarction, nonfatal stroke, coronary revascularization, and unstable angina in "time-to-event analysis."

Results

- 70.7% enrolled patients were in the secondary prevention cohort, while 29.3% of enrolled patients were in the primary prevention cohort.
- Median change in triglyceride level from baseline to 1 year was −18.3% (39.0 mg/dL) in icosapent ethyl group, while the placebo group had an increase in 2.2% (4.5 mg/dL).
- Primary endpoint events occurred in 17.2% of icosapent ethyl group vs. 22.0% of placebo group. To prevent one primary endpoint event, the number needed to treat was 21 patients over 4.9 years.
- Attaining a triglyceride level <150 mg/dL did not significantly decrease cardiovascular events.
- The overall rate of serious adverse events was low in both groups.
  - Bleeding events did occur more in the icosapent ethyl group, though there were no fatal bleeding episodes.
  - The rates of atrial fibrillation and peripheral edema were significant in the icosapent ethyl group compared to placebo at 5.3% vs. 3.9% and 6.5% vs. 5.0%.

Importance

The REDUCE-IT trial shows that icosapent ethyl (2 g twice daily) when used in combination with statin therapy can reduce the incidence of cardiovascular death, nonfatal myocardial infarction, nonfatal stroke, coronary revascularization, and unstable angina in patients with hypertriglyceridemia.

It should be noted that the authors of the study maintain that icosapent ethyl is structurally different than other formulations of fish oils and caution against generalizing the results of this study.

Bottom Line

Icosapent ethyl at a dose of 2 g twice daily in combination with statin therapy should be considered for primary and secondary preventions of cardiovascular events in patients with hypertriglyceridemia. It is effective at lowering triglyceride levels and decreases risk of cardiovascular events by 25%.

References

1. Ganda OP, Bhatt DL, Mason RP, Miller M, Boden WE. Unmet need for adjunctive dyslipidemia therapy in hypertriglyceridemia management. J Am Coll Cardiol. 2018;72(3):330–43. https://doi.org/10.1016/j.jacc.2018.04.061.

Part VII
Nephrology

Tracey Roesing

Chapter 39
ACE Inhibitors Impact on Slowing the Progression of Diabetic Nephropathy-1993

Tina Chuong

Background

The diabetes epidemic has caused diabetic nephropathy to become an important cause of chronic kidney disease and end-stage renal disease (ESRD) [1]. Diabetic nephropathy is characterized by albuminuria, increased arterial blood pressure, decline in glomerular filtration rate, and increased risk of cardiovascular morbidity and mortality [2]. This study was one of the first designed to evaluate the effects of angiotensin-converting-enzyme (ACE) inhibitors on diabetic nephropathy independent of blood pressure reduction.

Objective

- To determine whether an ACE inhibitor (captopril) is renoprotective, independent of blood pressure reduction, slowing the progression of diabetic nephropathy.

Lewis EJ, Hunsicker LG, Bain RP, Rodhe RD, et al. The Effect of Angiotensin-Converting-Enzyme Inhibition on Diabetic Nephropathy. N Engl J Med 1993;329:1456–1462.
Hyperlink to PDF: https://www.nejm.org/doi/pdf/10.1056/NEJM199311113292004?articleTools=true

---

T. Chuong (✉)
Jefferson Health, Abington, PA, USA

J. Russell, N. S. Skolnik (eds.), *Top Articles in Primary Care*,
https://doi.org/10.1007/978-3-031-25620-2_39

Design and Methods

- This study was a prospective, double-blind, randomized clinical trial performed in 30 centers.
  - Included 409 patients aged 18–49 who had insulin-dependent diabetes mellitus for at least 7 years, diabetic retinopathy, urinary protein excretion ≥500 mg per 24 h, and a serum creatinine concentration of ≤2.5 mg/dL.
- Study patients were divided into two groups: Captopril (25 mg three times a day) or Placebo (three times a day) with blood pressure goal of <140/90.
- Primary study end point was a doubling of baseline serum creatinine.
- Secondary end points included death, dialysis, transplantation, and changes in renal function.

Results

- Captopril significantly reduced the rate of renal function loss and this was not related to its antihypertensive effect. Serum creatinine doubled in 12.3% of the patients in the captopril group vs. 21.2% in the placebo group ($p = 0.007$), representing an approximately 48% reduction in the doubling of serum creatinine over 3 years.
- The effect was greatest in those with the highest creatinine at baseline.
- Captopril treatment showed a reduction in the composite outcome of death, dialysis, and transplantation by 50% compared to placebo.
- The effect of adding captopril was apparent within 6 months of starting the medication.

Importance

This trial played a major role in demonstrating the ability of ACE inhibitors to reduce the progression of albuminuria and decline in renal function in patients with insulin-dependent diabetes, independent of blood pressure reductions. Therefore, this suggested that providers consider the use of ACE inhibitors in normotensive or hypertensive patients with diabetic nephropathy. Prior to this study, only animal studies demonstrated the benefits of ACE inhibitors on reducing glomerular injury compared to other antihypertensive medications.

Updates

- Today, the American Diabetes Association (ADA) recommends ACE inhibitors or angiotensin receptor blockers (ARB) as first-line treatment for hypertensive diabetic patients with urinary albumin-to-creatinine ratio ≥300 mg/g creatinine or 30–299 mg/g creatinine (modest elevations). It is important to note that the ADA does not recommend ACE inhibitors or ARBs for patients without hypertension to prevent the development of diabetic kidney disease since no clinical trials have been performed to determine whether it would improve renal outcomes [3].

Bottom Line

- ACE inhibitors, like captopril are renoprotective and should be considered as a first-line medication in patients with diabetes, hypertension, and diabetic kidney disease.

References

1. Lim AKH. Diabetic nephropathy – complications and treatment. Int J Nephrol Renovasc Dis. 2014;7:361–81.
2. Hovind P, Rossing P, Tarnow L, Smidth U, et al. Progression of diabetic nephropathy. Kidney Int. 2001;59(2):702–9.
3. American Diabetes Association. Standards of medical Care in Diabetes – 2018 abridged for primary care providers. Clin Diabetes. 2018;36(1):14–37.

Chapter 40
ARB and the Slowing of Progression of Diabetic Nephropathy 2001

Sharon Buchbinder

Background

Diabetic nephropathy is a leading cause of end-stage renal disease worldwide [1]. When it was discovered that blocking the renin angiotensin system can have a renoprotective effect, research was initiated to study these effects using medications such as angiotensin-II-receptor antagonists (ARBs) and angiotensin converting enzyme (ACE) inhibitors in patients with type 1 diabetic nephropathy. Although type 2 is the most common form of diabetes, it was not until later that there was research on the renoprotective effects of medications for this population [1]. This study advanced the field by studying the effect of ARBs on type 2 diabetic nephropathy.

Brenner, B. M., Cooper, M. E., de Zeeuw, D., Keane, W. F., Mitch, W. E., Parving, H. H., Remuzzi, G., Snapinn, S. M., Zhang, Z., Shahinfar, S., & RENAAL Study Investigators (2001). Effects of Losartan on Renal and Cardiovascular Outcomes in Patients with Type 2 Diabetes and Nephropathy. *The New England journal of medicine*, *345*(12), 861–869.
Hyperlink to PDF: https://www.nejm.org/doi/10.1056/NEJMoa011161?url_ver=Z39.88-2003&rfr_id=ori:rid:crossref.org&rfr_dat=cr_pub%20%200www.ncbi.nlm.nih.gov

---

S. Buchbinder (✉)
Jefferson Health, Abington, PA, USA
e-mail: sharon.buchbinder@jefferson.edu

J. Russell, N. S. Skolnik (eds.), *Top Articles in Primary Care*, https://doi.org/10.1007/978-3-031-25620-2_40

Objective

- To determine whether losartan, an angiotensin-II-receptor antagonist (ARB), is renoprotective and cardioprotective for patients with type 2 diabetic nephropathy.
- The primary outcome was the combination of a doubling of the baseline serum creatinine concentration, end-stage renal disease (ESRD), and death.
- Secondary outcomes included morbidity and mortality from cardiovascular causes, the development of proteinuria, and rate of progression of renal disease.

Design and Methods

- One thousand five hundred thirteen patients with type 2 diabetes and nephropathy from 250 centers in 28 countries were enrolled in a randomized, double-blind study and placed in either an experimental group or placebo group.
- The experimental group received Losartan 50 or 100 mg daily. All patients in the experimental group were initially started on 50 mg and then after 4 weeks, if the patient's systolic blood pressure was >140 or the diastolic blood pressure was >90, the patient's dose was increased to Losartan 100 mg.
- Nephropathy was defined as having a urinary albumin/creatinine ratio > 300 or at least 0.5 g/day of protein and a serum creatinine between 1.3 and 3 mg/dL.
- The mean follow-up time of the study was 3.4 years.

Results

- Treatment with losartan reduced the risk of primary outcome including end points of doubling of the serum creatinine, ESRD, and death by 16% ($P = 0.02$).

Treatment with losartan reduced the risk of doubling serum creatinine by 25% ($P = 0.006$).

- Treatment with losartan reduced the risk of ESRD by 28% ($P = 0.002$).
- Treatment with losartan reduced the risk of proteinuria by 35% ($P < 0.001$).
- Treatment with losartan reduced the rate of first hospitalization for heart failure by 32% ($P = 0.005$).
- There were no significant differences in the rates of cardiovascular mortality and morbidity between the experimental and placebo group.

Importance

The RENAAL study demonstrated that Losartan (ARBs) significantly reduced the risk of doubling of serum creatinine and progression to ESRD, significantly lowered the levels of proteinuria and slowed the rate of decline in glomerular filtration rate in type 2 diabetics with nephropathy [2]. The ADA Standards of Medical Care in Diabetes included guidance that an ACE inhibitor or ARB is the recommended first-line treatment for hypertension in patients with diabetes and urinary albumin-to-creatinine ratio ≥ 300 mg/g creatinine (level of evidence: A) or 30–299 mg/g creatinine (level of evidence: B) [3].

Updates

- The IDNT study, published in 2001, showed that irbesartan slowed progression of nephropathy in type 2 diabetics, independent of its antihypertensive effect [4].
- The LIFE study, published in 2002, demonstrated that losartan did reduce the incidence of cardiovascular morbidity and mortality in hypertensive patients with diabetes and LVH [5].
- The MARVAL study, published in 2002, showed that valsartan lowered urine albumin excretion more effectively than amlodipine, independent of BP, in patients with type 2 diabetes [6].
- The INNOVATION study, published in 2007, demonstrated that telmisartan reduced the progression from microalbuminuria to macroalbuminuria and induced remission of microalbuminuria in patients with type 2 diabetes [7].
- The ROADMAP study, published in 2011, showed that olmesartan delayed the onset of microalbuminuria in patients with type 2 diabetes [8].

Bottom Line

- The RENAAL Study demonstrated that Losartan has renoprotective effects for patients with type 2 diabetic nephropathy and can delay the progression of renal disease and renal failure.

References

1. Mallik R, Chowdhury TA. Pharmacotherapy to delay the progression of diabetic kidney disease in people with type 2 diabetes: past, present and future. Ther Adv Endocrinol Metab. 2022;13:20420188221081601.
2. Rayner B. Advances in the treatment of diabetic renal disease: focus on losartan. Curr Med Res Opin. 2004;20(3):333–40.
3. American Diabetes Association. Microvascular complications and foot care. Sec. 9. In standards of medical Care in Diabetes 2016. Diabetes Care. 2016;39(Suppl. 1):S72–80.
4. Lewis EJ, Hunsicker LG, Clarke WR, Berl T, Pohl MA, Lewis JB, Ritz E, Atkins RC, Rohde R, Raz I, Collaborative Study Group. Renoprotective effect of the angiotensin-receptor antagonist irbesartan in patients with nephropathy due to type 2 diabetes. N Engl J Med. 2001;345(12):851–60.
5. Sica DA, Weber M. The losartan intervention for endpoint reduction (LIFE) trial-have angiotensin-receptor blockers come of age? J Clin Hypertens (Greenwich). 2002;4(4):301–5.
6. Viberti G, Wheeldon NM, MicroAlbuminuria Reduction With VALsartan (MARVAL) Study Investigators. Microalbuminuria reduction with valsartan in patients with type 2 diabetes mellitus: a blood pressure-independent effect. Circulation. 2002;106(6):672–8.
7. Makino H, Haneda M, Babazono T, Moriya T, Ito S, Iwamoto Y, Kawamori R, Takeuchi M, Katayama S, INNOVATION Study Group. Prevention of transition from incipient to overt nephropathy with telmisartan in patients with type 2 diabetes. Diabetes Care. 2007;30(6):1577–8.
8. Haller H, Viberti GC, Mimran A, Remuzzi G, Rabelink AJ, Ritz E, Rump LC, Ruilope LM, Katayama S, Ito S, Izzo JL Jr, Januszewicz A. Preventing microalbuminuria in patients with diabetes: rationale and design of the randomised Olmesartan and diabetes microalbuminuria prevention (ROADMAP) study. J Hypertens. 2006;24(2):403–8.

Chapter 41
SGLT2 Inhibitors and Diabetic Renal Protection-2020

Evan R. Gooberman

Background

Chronic kidney disease (CKD) affects millions of people worldwide and is a significant contributor to morbidity and mortality [1]. Angiotensin-converting enzyme (ACE) inhibitors and angiotensin II receptor blockers (ARBs) have been the primary medications available to provide renal protection [2]. Recently, SGLT2 inhibitors have been shown to reduce the risk of kidney failure in patients with type 2 diabetes [3].

Objective

- To determine the effect of dapagliflozin in patients with chronic kidney disease, with or without type 2 diabetes.
- Primary end points were sustained decline in eGFR of at least 50%, end-stage kidney disease, and death from renal or cardiovascular causes.
- Secondary end points were hospitalization for heart failure, death from cardiovascular causes, and death from any cause.

Heerspink HJL, Wheeler DC, et al. Dapagliflozin in Patients with Chronic Kidney Disease. N Engl J Med 2020; 383:1436–1446.
Hyperlink to article: https://www.nejm.org/doi/full/10.1056/NEJMoa2024816

E. R. Gooberman (✉)
Jefferson Health, Abington, PA, USA

J. Russell, N. S. Skolnik (eds.), *Top Articles in Primary Care*,
https://doi.org/10.1007/978-3-031-25620-2_41

Design and Methods

- Four thousand three hundred and four patients with an estimated glomerular filtration rate (eGFR) of 25–75 mL/min per 1.73 m^2 of body-surface area and a urinary albumin-to-creatinine ratio of 200–5000 were randomized in a double-blind trial.
- Randomization was monitored to ensure that at least 30% of the patients in each arm of the trial had type 2 diabetes and at least 30% of the patients in each arm of the trial did not have diabetes.
- Patients were required to be on an ACE inhibitor or ARB for at least 4 weeks prior to being assigned to one of two groups: 10 mg dapagliflozin daily or placebo daily.
- Patients were evaluated every 4 months for 2.0–2.7 years (2.4-year median). The independent data monitoring committee recommended ending the trial early due to efficacy based on 408 primary outcome events. At that point, all participants returned for a final study visit—4289 patients (99.7%) completed the trial.
- Data was evaluated based on the intention-to-treat population using a Cox proportional-hazards regression model with stratification according to the factors used at randomization.

Results

- Patients in the dapagliflozin group had 197/2152 (9.2%) primary outcome events occur compared to 312/2152 (14.5%) primary outcome events in the placebo group—the hazard ratio was 0.61 with a confidence interval of 0.51–0.72 ($p < 0.001$).
- The number needed to treat to prevent one primary outcome event was 19 (confidence interval of 15–27).
- The incidence of adverse events and serious adverse events was similar in the dapagliflozin group compared to the placebo group—there were no cases of diabetic ketoacidosis or Fournier's gangrene in the dapagliflozin group.

Importance

For decades, the only medications available to reduce the risk of chronic kidney disease progression have been ACE inhibitors and ARBs. The CREDENCE trial showed SGLT2 inhibitors may benefit patients with type 2 diabetes who have CKD [3]. With the DAPA-CKD trial, there is now evidence to show that effects of dapagliflozin on CKD outcomes were similar in patients with type 2 diabetes and in patients without type 2 diabetes.

Bottom Line

- Dapagliflozin (representing SGLT2 inhibitors) improves outcomes for patients with chronic kidney disease, regardless of the presence of type 2 diabetes.
- Note that Dapagliflozin was used safely in this trial in patients entering the trial with eGFR down to 25 mL/min per 1.73 m^2 of body-surface area.
- SGLT2 inhibitors should be considered for patients with chronic kidney disease and albuminuria, regardless of whether a patient has type 2 diabetes, to slow the rate of progression of CKD.

References

1. GBD Chronic Kidney Disease Collaboration. Global, regional, and national burden of chronic kidney disease, 1990-2017: a systematic analysis for the Global Burden of Disease Study 2017. Lancet. 2020;395:709–33.
2. Maschio G, Zuchelli P, et al. Effect of the angiotensin-converting enzyme inhibitor benazepril on the progression of chronic renal disease. N Engl J Med. 1996;334:939–45.
3. Perkovic P, Capuano G, et al. Canagliflozin and renal outcomes in type 2 diabetes and nephropathy. N Engl J Med. 2019;380:2295–306.

Chapter 42
Finerenone on Chronic Kidney Disease Outcomes in Type 2 Diabetes-2020

Rui Song

Background

Type 2 diabetes accounts for more than 90% of the 37 million people with diabetes in the United States [1] and is the leading cause of chronic kidney disease (CKD). Patients with diabetic nephropathy have a higher prevalence of cardiovascular (CV) disease and a higher risk of CKD progression than the general population [2]. Mild hyperaldosteronism is often found in patients with CKD and could lead to inflammation and fibrosis [2]. During its development, finerenone, a nonsteroidal selective mineralocorticoid receptor antagonist (MRA), showed renoprotective effects in diabetes [3]. FIDELIO-DKD trial investigated the long-term effects of finerenone on CKD outcomes in patients with type 2 diabetes.

Objectives

- To compare finerenone with placebo, with regard to renal and CV outcomes in patients with CKD and type 2 diabetes.
- Primary outcomes were kidney failure (defined as renal dialysis or transplantation, at least 40% eGFR decline from baseline, or eGFR < 15 mL/min) or death.

Bakris GL, Agarwal R, Anker SD, et al. Effect of Finerenone on Chronic Kidney Disease Outcomes in Type 2 Diabetes. N Eng J Med 2020; 383:2219–2229.
Hyperlink to PDF: https://www.nejm.org/doi/full/10.1056/NEJMoa2025845

R. Song (✉)
Jefferson Health, Abington, PA, USA
e-mail: Rui.song@jefferson.edu

J. Russell, N. S. Skolnik (eds.), *Top Articles in Primary Care*,
https://doi.org/10.1007/978-3-031-25620-2_42

- Key secondary outcomes included CV death, non-fatal myocardial infarction, nonfatal stroke, or hospitalization for heart failure.

Design and Methods

- This double-blind, multicenter trial recruited 5734 patients with CKD and type 2 diabetes and randomly assigned them to either a finerenone or a placebo group.
- Inclusion criteria were microalbuminuria (urinary albumin-to-creatinine ratio, UACR, 30–300 mg/g) with an eGFR 25–60 mL/min/1.73 m^2 and diabetic retinopathy or gross albuminuria (UACR 300–5000 mg/g) with an eGFR 25–75 mL/min/1.73 m^2.
- All patients used the maximum tolerated dose of renin-angiotensin system (RAS) blockade with baseline serum potassium levels ≤4.8 mmol/L.
- Median follow-up time of the study was 2.6 years (2015–2018).

Results

- Finerenone had a significantly lower incidence of the primary composite outcome of kidney failure (dialysis, transplantation, or eGFR <15 mL/min), a sustained reduction of at least 40% in the eGFR from baseline, or death from renal causes than the placebo group. The primary outcome occurred in 17.8% in the finerenone group and 21.1% in the placebo group with a hazard ratio of 0.82 ($P = 0.001$).
- Finerenone had a significantly lower risk of the key secondary outcome of CV complications including CV death, nonfatal myocardial infarction, nonfatal stroke, or hospitalization for heart failure, compared with the placebo group—13.0% vs. 14.8% in the respective groups with a hazard ratio of 0.86 ($P = 0.03$).
- Finerenone was associated with a 31% greater reduction in the UACR than placebo.
- The finerenone group had a higher incidence of hyperkalemia (18.3%) than the placebo group (9%), though only 2.3% of patients with hyperkalemia needed to discontinue finerenone.

Importance

Previous clinical strategies to prevent CV disease and progression of CKD in the diabetic population for the past three decades include a limited number of medications—angiotensin-converting-enzyme inhibitors (ACEi), angiotensin-receptor blockers (ARB), and, most recently, sodium-glucose cotransporter 2 (SGLT-2) inhibitors. The blockage of multiple targets in the RAS has been attractive to researchers aiming to maximize the beneficial effects of RAS inhibition. However, results from the trials with dual inhibition with ACEi plus ARB or direct renin inhibitors were disappointing [4, 5]. The FIDELIO-DKD trial chose the downstream target of RAS, the aldosterone receptor, for an attempt at demonstrating beneficial effects on renal and CV disease.

It is well established that spironolactone and eplerenone, both steroidal MRAs, are beneficial in patients with CV disease [2]. Finerenone, a nonsteroidal MRA, has a lower risk of hyperkalemia and thus was chosen for this CKD trial with combination use of ACEi/ARB [2]. In fact, discontinuation of finerenone due to hyperkalemia was infrequent (2.3%) and was markedly less frequent than in trials of dual RAS blockade [4, 5].

The FIDELIO-DKD trial demonstrated the efficacy of finerenone in treating patients with type 2 diabetes and stage 3–4 CKD with respect to both renal and CV benefits. It is the first large phase 3 randomized trial assessing the long-term effects of MRA in DKD and proved that controlling relative hyperaldosteronism in patients with DKD is a promising strategy.

Updates

- In 2021, the FIGARO-DKD trial [6] again showed lower kidney and CV events in those patients treated with finerenone than those treated with placebo, highlighting the importance of early intervention in diabetic patients with mild-to-moderate CKD in order to prevent CV events.
- The FDA approved finerenone in treating adults with CKD and type 2 diabetes in July 2021.
- In an update to the American Diabetes Association's Standards of Care in May 2022 [7], the standards were updated to say, "For patients with type 2 diabetes and chronic kidney disease treated with maximum tolerated doses of ACE inhibitors or angiotensin receptor blockers, addition of finerenone should be considered to improve cardiovascular outcomes and reduce the risk of chronic kidney disease progression. A."

Bottom Line

- Finerenone should be considered for patients with diabetes and CKD, with close monitoring for the development of hyperkalemia.

References

1. https://www.cdc.gov/diabetes/data/statistics-report/. Accessed 26 March 2022.
2. Ingelfinger JR, Rosen CJ. Finerenone - halting relative hyperaldosteronism in chronic kidney disease. N Engl J Med. 2020;383:2285–6.
3. Bakris GL, Agarwal R, Chan JC, et al. Effect of finerenone on albuminuria in patients with diabetic nephropathy: a randomized clinical trial. JAMA. 2015;314:884–94.
4. Parving H-H, Brenner BM, McMurray JJV, et al. Cardiorenal end points in a trial of aliskiren for type 2 diabetes. N Engl J Med. 2012;367:2204–13.
5. Imai E, Chan JCN, Ito S, et al. Effects of olmesartan on renal and cardiovascular outcomes in type 2 diabetes with overt nephropathy: a multicentre, randomised, placebo-controlled study. Diabetologia. 2011;54:2978–86.
6. Pitt B, Filippatos G, Agarwal R, et al. Cardiovascular events with finerenone in kidney disease and type 2 diabetes. N Engl J Med. 2021;385:2252–63.
7. American Diabetes Association Standards of Care. Addendum. 2022. https://diabetesjournals.org/care/article/doi/10.2337/dc22-ad08/147053/Addendum-10-Cardiovascular-Disease-and-Risk.

Part VIII
Obesity

Samantha Flanagan

Chapter 43
Phen/Fen for Weight Loss-1984

Angela Kalinowski

Background

It has been shown that there are important differences between fenfluramine hydrochloride and the traditional stimulant drugs used in treating obesity. The stimulant anorexiants are believed to act via central catecholamine mechanisms whereas fenfluramine appears to act via serotonergic mechanisms. The traditional stimulant drugs have adverse effects including insomnia, nervousness, increased motor activity, and occasional cardiovascular disturbances including increased pulse rate and increased blood pressure. They also appear to delay the onset of eating and to shorten its duration. Fenfluramine often causes sedative effects and occasionally diarrhea.

Objective

To see if the differences between available anorexiants could be utilized to create a treatment regimen with maintained efficacy but fewer side effects therefore improving long-term acceptance of treatment.

Weintraub, M., Hasday, J., Mushlin, A., & Lockwood, D. (1984). A double-blind clinical trial in weight control. Use of fenfluramine and phentermine alone and in combination. *Archives of Internal Medicine*, *144*(6), 1143–1148. doi: 10.1001/archinte.144.6.1143
https://jamanetwork.com/journals/jamainternalmedicine/article-abstract/604539

A. Kalinowski (✉)
Jefferson Health, Abington, PA, USA
e-mail: angeladibileo@gmsail.com

J. Russell, N. S. Skolnik (eds.), *Top Articles in Primary Care*,
https://doi.org/10.1007/978-3-031-25620-2_43

Design and Methods

- The researchers performed a controlled clinical trial using a double-blind, parallel-group design comparing phentermine (delayed release), 30 mg in the morning; fenfluramine hydrochloride, 20 mg three times a day; placebo; and a combination of phentermine, 15 mg in the morning; and fenfluramine hydrochloride, 30 mg before the evening meal.
- Patients received placebos as needed to ensure that all patients received three doses every day.
- The schedule encompassed a 3-week run-in period of diet only, 16 weeks of drug treatment plus diet, 4 weeks of tapering the medication, and finally 4 weeks of follow-up without medication.
- The 81 participants were 18–55 years of age and 130–180% of their ideal body. They were not taking any other medications and did not have diabetes mellitus, hypertension, or hyperlipidemia.
- Five dietitians devised individualized balanced diets based on participant preferences, calculated at 20 kcal/kg of ideal body weight. Dietitians also discussed basic techniques of eating behavior modification with the participants at weeks 1, 6, and 20.
- Participants were assigned a blinded study physician. At clinic visits weights were measured and discussed. Compliance was assessed by questioning the participants and by counting the unused capsules. Participants marked estimates of their hunger and their degree of fullness experienced on a visual analogue scale. Adverse effects were assessed through both open-ended questions and the use of a predetermined checklist.
- Weight loss was corrected for initial weight by use of the Feinstein Reduction Index (FRI).
- FRI = $(W_{\text{initial}}/W_{\text{ideal}}) \times (W_{\text{loss}}/W_{\text{initial}} - W_{\text{ideal}}) \times 100$ where W represents weight. A higher FRI indicates greater weight loss.

Results

- At all time points, beginning at week 6, active treatment participants lost significantly more weight than those receiving placebo.
- The percentage of weight loss from baseline for the active treatment groups was statistically significantly greater than that for the placebo group.
- The participants receiving the three active treatments had higher FRI scores (indicating greater weight loss) than did the placebo-treated participants.
- Participants receiving the combination and phentermine had hunger ratings below baseline values throughout the study.
- In the combination group, there was an increase in fullness ratings.

- Patients in the phentermine and fenfluramine groups had statistically significantly more complaints than those receiving placebo.
- There was no significant difference between combination and placebo or between the three active treatments in total complaints. However, combination group participants reported significantly fewer cardiovascular and CNS complaints than the phentermine participants.
- Both the phentermine and the fenfluramine group had statistically more cardiovascular and CNS complaints than the placebo group. Again, there was no significant difference between combination and placebo.
- No participant on the combination complained of palpitations, although several participants in the other treatment groups did so.
- A smaller percentage of the participants remaining in the study receiving the combination had any complaint compared with participants receiving phentermine or fenfluramine alone.

Importance

In this placebo-controlled, double-blind clinical trial, a combination of half doses of a stimulant anorexiant and fenfluramine was as effective as full doses of the individual medications and more effective than placebo. The participants receiving this combination had fewer adverse effects and less hunger and increased fullness. Individualized diets and some behavior modification techniques were both reinforced during the study. Therefore, it was demonstrated that appetite control medications could be more effective. This study showed these medications could produce more sustained weight loss. They were previously only thought to temporarily cause weight loss. A very small study led to a huge amount of use for these medications for weight loss across the nation.

Updates

- In a study published in the *New England Journal of Medicine* in 1997, it was found that patients evaluated about a year after starting combination phentermine and fenfluramine therapy demonstrated unusual valvular morphology and regurgitation on echocardiography. Both right sided and left-sided heart valves were involved. Some patients also had newly documented pulmonary hypertension [1].
- At the time of this study, there were 18 million prescriptions for combination therapy [1].
- In 1997, fenfluramine was recalled by the FDA after continued reports that it caused heart valve defects [2].

Bottom Line

Combining fenfluramine and phentermine capitalized on their pharmacodynamic differences, resulting in equivalent weight loss, fewer adverse effects, and better appetite control. However, in 1997 fenfluramine was recalled after studies showed that it caused heart valve defects.

References

1. Connolly H, et al. Valvular heart disease associated with fenfluramine–phentermine. N Engl J Med. 1997;337(24):1772–6. https://doi.org/10.1056/nejm199712113372414.
2. Anti-obesity drugs recalled from global market. Lancet. 1997;350(9081):867. https://doi.org/10.1016/s0140-6736(97)23038-2.

Chapter 44
Semaglutide in Obesity (STEP-1 Trial)-2021

Samantha P. Flanagan

Background

Obesity is a global and national health concern that is costly and growing in prevalence. From 2017 to March 2020 an estimated 41.9% of Americans were obese [1]. Obesity increases the risk of many conditions including type 2 diabetes, stroke, heart disease, and certain cancers. The STEP-1 trial investigated the effectiveness of semaglutide 2.4 mg in helping adults with obesity achieve weight loss.

Objective

- To evaluate the efficacy of semaglutide 2.4 mg as an adjunct to lifestyle modifications in reducing body weight in patients with overweight or obesity without diabetes.

Wilding JP, Batterham RL, et al. Once-weekly semaglutide in adults with overweight or obesity. New England Journal of Medicine 2021; 385(1).
Hyperlink to PDF: https://www.nejm.org/doi/pdf/10.1056/NEJMoa2032183?articleTools=true

S. P. Flanagan (✉)
Main Line Health, King of Prussia, PA, USA

J. Russell, N. S. Skolnik (eds.), *Top Articles in Primary Care*, https://doi.org/10.1007/978-3-031-25620-2_44

Design and Methods

- This study was a randomized, double-blind, placebo-controlled trial of 1961 participants in 16 countries and 129 sites.
- Participants included patients 18 and older with at least one self-reported attempt to lose weight without success and a BMI of 30 or greater or a BMI of 27 or greater with at least one weight-related comorbidity.
- The study excluded those with diabetes defined as a glycated hemoglobin level (hemoglobin A1c) of 6.5% or greater.
- Patients received semaglutide 2.4 mg for 68 weeks, doses began at 0.25 mg weekly and were increased every 4 weeks until reaching the maximum dosage of 2.4 mg at week 16.
- In addition to medication, patients received individual counseling sessions every 4 weeks to help them achieve a 500-kcal deficit per day and increased physical activity.
- Primary endpoints were percentage change in body weight from baseline and achievement of a reduction in body weight of more than 5%.
- Data was evaluated with an intention-to-treat analysis.

Results

- The mean weight change at week 68 was -14.9% in the semaglutide group compared with -2.4% in the placebo group.
- 86.4% of participants in the treatment group lost at least 5% of their body weight.
- Gastrointestinal side effects were most commonly reported and occurred more frequently in the treatment group at 74.2% and 47.9% respectively.

Importance

The STEP 1 trial represents a major development in the treatment of obesity as a disease. The use of once-weekly semaglutide helps patients achieve greater weight loss than lifestyle interventions alone and compared to any other FDA-approved medication for weight loss to date. The ease of use, safety, and efficacy of semaglutide make it a popular choice for patients and providers.

Updates

- Since the STEP 1 trial there have been subsequent studies (STEP 2–8).

- STEP 2 examined semaglutide 2.4 mg in patients with overweight or obesity and diabetes showing statistically significant weight loss compared to placebo. Diabetics had been excluded from the STEP 1 trial [2].
- STEP 4 examined continuation of semaglutide versus discontinuation after 20 weeks of therapy finding that continued use resulted in greater weight loss compared to placebo [3].
- STEP 8 compared daily liraglutide 3.0 mg and weekly semaglutide 2.4 mg head-to-head finding a statistically greater weight loss with semaglutide compared to liraglutide. Mean body weight loss was 15.8% and 6.4% respectively [4].

Bottom Line

- Semaglutide 2.4 mg is an effective adjunct to lifestyle modification in the treatment of overweight and obesity.
- At the time of this publication, semaglutide 2.4 mg is the most effective FDA approved medication for the treatment of weight loss.

References

1. US Department of Health and Human Services. Adult obesity facts. Centers for Disease Control and Prevention. 2022. https://www.cdc.gov/obesity/data/adult.html. Accessed 18 May 2022.
2. Davies M, Færch L, Jeppesen OK, Pakseresht A, Pedersen SD, Perreault L, Rosenstock J, Shimomura I, Viljoen A, Wadden TA, Lingvay I. Semaglutide 2·4 mg once a week in adults with overweight or obesity, and type 2 diabetes (step 2): a randomized, double-blind, double-dummy, placebo-controlled, phase 3 trial. Lancet. 2021;397:971–84.
3. Rubino D, Abrahamsson N, Davies M, Hesse D, Greenway FL, Jensen C, Lingvay I, Mosenzon O, Rosenstock J, Rubio MA, Rudofsky G, Tadayon S, Wadden TA, Dicker D, Friberg M, Sjödin A, Dicker D, Segal G, Mosenzon O, et al. Effect of continued weekly subcutaneous semaglutide vs placebo on weight loss maintenance in adults with overweight or obesity. JAMA. 2021;325(14):1414.
4. Rubino DM, Greenway FL, Khalid U, O'Neil PM, Rosenstock J, Sørrig R, Wadden TA, Wizert A, Garvey WT, Arauz-Pacheco C, Cannon K, Downey HJ, Fitz-Patrick D, Geohas J, Gerety G, Gilbert J, Hollander P, Klein E, Laufer K, et al. Effect of weekly subcutaneous semaglutide vs daily liraglutide on body weight in adults with overweight or obesity without diabetes. JAMA. 2022;327(2):138.

Chapter 45
Carbohydrate-Insulin Model for Obesity-2021

Samantha P. Flanagan

Background

Obesity affects over 40% of Americans, a percentage that has been steadily climbing despite public health guidance to "eat less and move more." Obesity increases the risk of many of the leading causes of preventable death including heart disease and type 2 diabetes [1]. This perspective piece explores an alternative model, the carbohydrate-insulin model (CIM) compared to the energy balance model (EBM).

Objective

- To compare the carbohydrate-insulin model (CIM) of obesity to the widely accepted energy balance model (EBM) of obesity.

Design, Methods, and Definitions

- This perspective piece uses currently available literature to explore the difference between the EBM and CIM models.

Ludwig, DS, Aronne, LJ, et al. *The carbohydrate-insulin model. A physiological perspective on the obesity pandemic. The American Journal of Clinical Nutrition 2021, 114(6), 1873–1885.*
Hyperlink to PDF: https://academic.oup.com/ajcn/article/114/6/1873/6369073

S. P. Flanagan (✉)
Main Line Health, King of Prussia, PA, USA

J. Russell, N. S. Skolnik (eds.), *Top Articles in Primary Care*,
https://doi.org/10.1007/978-3-031-25620-2_45

- Energy Balance Model: Considers obesity a disorder of energy balance exacerbated by readily available and highly palatable, energy dense foods and compounded by sedentary lifestyle.
- Carbohydrate-Insulin Model: Argues that obesity is a result of a dysregulated hormonal and metabolic response to high glycemic load carbohydrates in the diet.

Results

- Both models assume that changes in food quality drive weight gain; however they differ in that the CIM model posits that metabolic responses to dietary calories and not simply calorie content are essential to understanding the disease of obesity.
- The CIM model attributes dietary glycemic load as a paramount driver of obesity.
- The CIM model proposes that by restricting carbohydrate intake a decrease in the insulin-to-glucagon ratio occurs, there is enhanced lipolysis and fat oxidation, and ultimately a lower intake of food.
- The consumption of high glycemic load foods including processed grains, potato products, and high sugar content foods causes increased insulin secretion, suppression of glucagon, and a glucose-dependent insulin otropic polypeptide also known as gastric inhibitory polypeptide (GIP) dominant incretin response leading to an anabolic state that increases glucose uptake in the muscle, liver, and adipose tissue.
- In the center of this model is insulin; as illustrated in this paper multiple studies have shown that the administration of exogenous insulin increases food intake and adiposity in both rodents and humans.
- Additionally, individuals with high insulin secretion or other derangements of glucose homeostasis are more susceptible to weight gain when consuming a high-glycemic load diet.
- If the CIM is correct, the negative energy balance model (EBM) defined by increased physical activity and decreased caloric intake will be unsuccessful in helping patients to achieve meaningful weight loss.

Importance

The carbohydrate-insulin model of obesity represents a paradigm change in the way science and medicine think about the disease of obesity. This perspective paper highlights just how early science and medicine are in understanding human metabolism and body weight regulation. Despite understanding only being in its early stages, this article uses currently available evidence to argue that the quality of our nutrition may be more important than the quantity of calories consumed.

Bottom Line

- Science and medicine have a long way to go in understanding the complex biological mechanisms behind obesity; however, the carbohydrate-insulin model serves as a promising alternative to the energy balance model in understanding and managing obesity by focusing on the quality of calories rather than the quantity consumed.

Reference

1. US Department of Health and Human Services. Adult obesity facts. Centers for Disease Control and Prevention. 2022. https://www.cdc.gov/obesity/data/adult.html. Accessed 18 May 2022.

Chapter 46
Tirzepatide for Obesity-2022

Christian Iversen

Background

Obesity is an increasingly common chronic disease associated with increased morbidity and mortality. Physiologic regulatory mechanisms limit the efficacy of diet and exercise to treat obesity once present, and both surgical and pharmacological treatments have been investigated to improve long-term management. Glucagon-like peptide-1 (GLP-1) and glucose-dependent insulinotropic peptide (GIP) are associated with insulin secretion and improved glucose tolerance and have been utilized for management of diabetes and weight loss. Tirzepatide is a co-agonist for GLP-1 and GIP receptors which has previously demonstrated improved glycemic improvement and weight loss when compared with a GLP-1 agonist (semaglutide). This randomized controlled trial studied the effect of tirzepatide for weight loss and other cardiometabolic measures.

Jastreboff, AM, Aronne, LJ, Ahmad, NN, Wharton S, Connery, L, Alves, B, Kiyosue, A, Zhang, S, Liu, B, Bunck, MC, & Stefanski, A for the SURMOUNT-1 investigators. (2022). Tirzepatide Once Weekly for the Treatment of Obesity. New England Journal of Medicine, 2022 June 4 (ahead of print). https://doi.org/10.1056/NEJMoa2206038
Hyperlink to PDF: https://www.nejm.org/doi/full/10.1056/NEJMoa2206038

C. Iversen (✉)
Jefferson Health, Abington, PA, USA
e-mail: Christian.iversen@jefferson.edu

J. Russell, N. S. Skolnik (eds.), *Top Articles in Primary Care*,
https://doi.org/10.1007/978-3-031-25620-2_46

Objective

- To assess the safety and efficacy of tirzepatide for weight loss and improvement of other cardiometabolic factors in people with obesity.

Design and Methods

- This was a multicenter, double-blind, placebo-controlled, randomized study enrolling adults with obesity or weight-related complications. 2539 participants were recruited, and the study was performed between December 2019 and April 2022.
- Key inclusion criteria: 18 years and older with a body mass index (BMI) over 30 or greater than 27 with a non-diabetic, weight-related complication (hypertension, dyslipidemia, obstructive sleep apnea, cardiovascular disease).
- Key exclusion criteria: diagnosis with diabetes, change in body weight more than 5 kg in 90 days before screening, previous or planned surgical treatment for obesity, or weight loss medications within 90 days of screening.
- Patients were randomly assigned in a 1:1:1:1 ratio to once-weekly subcutaneous injections of tirzepatide 5 mg, 10 mg, 15 mg, or placebo. Patients in the treatment arms started at 2.5 mg weekly with dose escalation of 2.5 mg every 4 weeks until the goal was achieved.
- Patients also received regular dietary/nutritional counseling and had goals of 500 calorie deficit per day from their daily estimated requirement and 150 min of physical activity weekly.
- All patients were followed for 72 weeks. Patients who were not prediabetic on initial screening were subsequently followed at 4 weeks from completion for safety assessment. Patients who had prediabetes on screening were enrolled for an additional 2-year trial period. The current study includes data from the 72-week study and 4-week follow-up.
- Primary endpoints were percentage change in body weight from baseline to week 72 and weight loss over 5%. Select secondary endpoints included change in weight at 20 weeks, change in cardiometabolic factors (waist circumference, systolic blood pressure, fasting insulin and lipid levels), and change in physical function score. A subgroup (~10%) of patients received body-fat mass assessment by dual-energy x-ray absorptiometry. Data was analyzed by intention-to-treat.

Results

- Demographics for the enrolled participants included: mean age 44.9 years, 67.5% female, 70.6% white, mean body weight 104.8 kg (231.0 lb), mean BMI 38.0, and mean weight circumference 114.1 cm. 94.5% had BMI greater than 30 and 40.6% had prediabetes.
- Of 2539 patients enrolled, 86.0% completed the 72-week study period, with higher completion in the treatment groups (88.4–89.8% in treatment groups vs 77.0% for placebo). There was 81.9% adherence to treatment or placebo. There was a higher discontinuation rate for adverse events in the tirzepatide groups compared to placebo (4.3–7.1% for treatment vs 2.6% for placebo).
- Mean change in weight at 72 weeks was −15.0%, −19.5%, −20.9% for 5-mg, 10-mg, and 15-mg tirzepatide doses, respectively. The mean weight change for the placebo for placebo group was −3.1%.
- Over 25% weight loss was achieved by 15%, 32%, and 36% of participants for 5-mg, 10-mg, and 15-mg tirzepatide doses, respectively. 1.5% of participants in the placebo group achieved over 25% weight loss.
- Treatment with tirzepatide positively impacted all measured cardiometabolic factors greater than placebo. Of patients with baseline prediabetes, 95% of the treatment group became normoglycemic compared with 62% of patients who received the placebo. Total body fat mass decreased by a mean of 33.9% with treatment compared to 8.2% for placebo.
- Side effects of tirzepatide were mostly mild to moderate and transient during the dose escalation period. Most commonly, these included nausea and diarrhea. Cholecystitis and acute cholecystitis were more common in the tirzepatide groups but had a low overall incidence (≤0.6%).

Importance

This study demonstrated the efficacy of tirzepatide, a co-agonist of GLP-1 and GIP, to promote weight loss and improvement in cardiometabolic markers with limited side effects. Importantly, participants had access to nutritional counseling, were instructed to maintain a 500 calorie daily deficit, and to exercise 150 minutes per week. The levels of weight loss achieved surpassed the widely recommended goal of 5–10% which have been shown to improve metabolic health. Mean weight loss was 15.0%, 19.5%, and 20.9% for 5-mg, 10-mg, and 15-mg doses of tirzepatide, respectively, compared with 3.1% for the placebo group. This study was limited to 72 weeks but will continue following patients for an additional 2 years to further assess outcomes.

Bottom Line

Patients treated with tirzepatide, a co-agonist of GLP-1 and GIP, in combination with lifestyle interventions including diet and exercise demonstrated significant weight loss and improvement of cardiometabolic factors with minimal side effects over the course of 72 weeks.

Part IX
Orthopaedics

Sean Carnahan

Chapter 47
Signs of Non-organic Back Pain-1980

Bree Zeyzus Johns

Background

Low back pain is a very common health problem with an estimated lifetime prevalence of 60–70% in industrialized countries [1]. It is also a major cause of disability. Low back pain is caused by a myriad of pathologies, and signs of organic causes of disease demonstrated in the physical exam support the diagnosis of pathology when present. Conversely, signs of nonorganic problems are findings that deviate from the usual presentation of disease. In the early 1900s, such signs were believed to be due to malingering or were used to identify patients with pain that is purely of a psychological basis. In their sentinel paper, Waddell et al. refuted this claim as an overly simplistic notion, and described a group of signs, "behavioral signs" or "inappropriate signs," that indicate the presence of coexisting nonorganic problems that contribute to disability from low back pain [1].

Objective

- To identify and classify physical signs that are incongruent with accepted patterns of low back pain pathology and that may warrant more comprehensive psychological evaluation.

Waddell, G., McCulloch, J.A., Kummel, E., & Venner, R.M. (1980). Nonorganic physical signs in low-back pain. *SPINE, 5*(2): 117-125. https://journals.lww.com/spinejournal/Abstract/1980/03000/Nonorganic_Physical_Signs_in_Low_Back_Pain.5.aspx

B. Zeyzus Johns (✉)
Jefferson Health, Abington, PA, USA

J. Russell, N. S. Skolnik (eds.), *Top Articles in Primary Care*,
https://doi.org/10.1007/978-3-031-25620-2_47

Design and Methods

- Four separate studies were conducted between two centers, located in Toronto, Canada, and Glasgow, Great Britain.
- Canadian patients (Study 1, $n = 84$; Study 2, $n = 50$) were mainly men with histories of chronic back pain and work loss over months to years and a high incidence of treatment failure but no psychiatric history, neurotic symptoms, or history of illness behavior.
- British patients (Study 3, $n = 100$; Study 4, $n = 70$) were both men and women with similar histories of prolonged pain, disability, and failed treatment but no psychiatric history, neurotic symptoms, or history of illness behavior.
- A fifth group of patients in the UK ($n = 50$) served as normal controls without back pain.
- Eight signs were grouped into five categories: tenderness, simulation, distraction, regional disturbances, and overreaction (Table 47.1).
- Reliability was shown with independent examinations by two observers in Study 2.
- Mean length of time between examinations (between two examiners) was 23 days.
- An additional 16 other signs were investigated, however, were not included in the final assessment due to poor inter- and intra-tester reliability, overlap with other signs, and difficulty for the examiner to execute.
- The presence of nonorganic signs observed during the physical exam was scored as positive and was correlated to scores on the hypochondriasis, depression, and hysteria scales of the Minnesota Multiphasic Personality Inventory (MMPI; measure of psychological distress in patients with low back pain).

Table 47.1 Wadell's Tests for Nonorganic Physical Signs

Test	Inappropriate Response[a]
Tenderness	Superficial, nonanatomic tenderness to touch
Simulation	
Axial loading	Vertical loading on a standing patient's skull produces low back pain
Rotation	Passive rotation of shoulders and pelvis in same plane causes low back pain
Distraction	Discrepancy between findings on sitting and supine straight leg raising tests
Regional disturbances	
Weakness	"Cogwheel" (give-way) weakness
Sensory	Nondermatomal sensory loss
Overreaction	Disproportionate facial expression, verbalization, or tremor during examination

[a]Three or more inappropriate responses suggest complicating psychosocial issues in patients with low back pain

- The presence of three or more types of nonorganic signs co-occurring with organic signs was considered a "positive Waddell's nonorganic signs test."
- The presence of only one or two nonorganic signs co-occurring with organic signs was considered a "negative Waddell's nonorganic signs test."

Results

- The scoring methodology was found to be highly reliable with 86% agreement between two examiners in detecting nonorganic signs.
- Objective findings including referred leg or root pain, relation of pain to time and activity, localized physical and radiologic findings of spinal abnormality, nerve root irritation or compression all showed no correlation to the nonorganic signs.
- Nonorganic signs were less common in patients with clear-cut pathology (fracture, congenital anomaly, deformity), and did not occur in control subjects.
- Nonorganic signs were unrelated to age, sex, or type of work.
- Overreaction was the most difficult to identify and required clinician judgment based on observation of behavior.
- Study 1 revealed a small correlation with the scoring on the MMPI when patients had three or more types of nonorganic signs, indicating psychological distress.

Importance

Psychological factors including behavioral, cognitive, or somatoform represent important contributors to chronic LBP and associated movement dysfunction. Wadell et al. were the first clinicians to define methods for the assessment of physical signs that are incongruent with typical patterns of pathology, and that point toward a nonphysiologic element of the patient's presentation. The Waddell tests consist of a set of five maneuvers easily performed during a routine physical examination that identify nonorganic factors that play an important role in persistent low back complaints. The presence of three or more inappropriate responses suggest complicating psychosocial issues and should not be construed as malingering as doing so would impede improvement in activity tolerance. Instead, patients should undergo more comprehensive psychological assessment and interventions should be implemented to target all contributing factors. Importantly, the authors stress how nonorganic signs frequently coexist with organic findings and the presence of one does not exclude or undermine the other. While Wadell et al. initially developed these signs to identify patients with low back pain likely to experience a poor surgical outcome, positive Wadell testing is now used to view back pain within a psychosocial context. Positive psychosocial signs should not be misinterpreted medico-legally, but instead should be viewed as important contributors to illness behavior and, therefore, to disability. Physical therapy should incorporate focused treatment to reduce the degree of disability and patients may benefit from further psychological testing and behavioral modification to address these elements of their pain. Since their original work, others have developed treatment-based classification schemes that incorporate nonorganic signs [2, 3]. Additionally, a US Agency for Health Care Policy and Research Clinical Practice Guideline from 1997 recommends exploring psychological factors when a patient with low back pain is having difficulty regaining activity tolerance [4].

Bottom Line

- Nonorganic factors can be important contributors to the symptoms of low back pain.
- As part of the physical exam, three or more Wadell's signs may detect a psychological component of low back pain and can be associated with symptom magnification, illness behavior, and disability.
- Psychological factors contributing to pain complaints and physical dysfunction should not be misconstrued as malingering but should prompt the clinician to recommend further psychological assessment.

References

1. World Health Organization. 2013. Priority methods for Europe and the world- 2013 update. https://www.who.int/medicines/areas/priority_medicines/MasterDocJune28_FINAL_Web.pdf.
2. Delitto A, Erhard RE, Boling RW. A treatment-based classification approach to low back syndrome: identifying and staging patients for conservative treatment. Phys Ther. 1995;75:470–89. https://doi.org/10.1093/ptj/75.6.470.
3. Marras WS, Parnianpour M, Ferguson SA, Kim JY, Crowell RR, Bose S, Simon SR. The classification of anatomic and symptom-based low back disorders using motion measure models. Spine. 1995;20(23):2531–46. https://doi.org/10.1097/00007632-199512000-00013.
4. Bigos S, Bowyer O, Braen G, Brown K, Deyo R, Haldeman S, et al. Acute low back problems in adults: clinical practice guideline No. 14. Rockville, MD: Agency for Health Care Policy and Research, Public Health Service, US Department of Health and Human Services; 1994. AHCPR, 95-0642. https://chiro.org/LINKS/GUIDELINES/Acute_Lower_Back_Problems_in_Adults.html.

Chapter 48
Ottawa Ankle Rules-X-Rays in Ankle Injuries-1992

Sean P. Carnahan

Background

Ankle fracture rate in acute injury (twisting, falls, direct blows, motor vehicle accidents) was shown to be less than 15%, yet radiographic assessment was typically the second most commonly performed musculoskeletal examination in the Emergency Department (ED) behind cervical-spine series.

Objective

- Develop a set of rules that would predict, with 100% sensitivity, fractures in acute ankle injury, in turn providing clinical reason and support for ordering radiographic assessment.

Stiell IG, Greenberg GH, McKnight RD, Nair RC, McDowell I, Worthington JR. A study to develop clinical decision rules for the use of radiography in acute ankle injuries. Annals of Emergency Medicine. 21 April 1992
Hyperlink to PDF:

S. P. Carnahan (✉)
UPMC, Pittsburgh, PA, USA
e-mail: carnahansp@upmc.edu

J. Russell, N. S. Skolnik (eds.), *Top Articles in Primary Care*,
https://doi.org/10.1007/978-3-031-25620-2_48

Design and Methods

- Prospective survey of 750 acute, blunt, ankle injury patients in Ottawa-based emergency departments was studied from July through December 1990.
- Multiple variables were used for the derivation of both ankle and foot radiographic series rules including patient age, mechanism of injury, physical exam findings, and ability to bear weight.

Results

- Developed 100% sensitive guidelines (Table 48.1)—no patient who had a negative for the rule would have a fracture.
- Provided physicians with the confidence to forego ankle and foot x-ray thus reducing costs without increasing likelihood of missing a fracture.

Table 48.1 This model represents the initial set of clinical decision rules

Ottawa Ankle Rules	
Clinical decision rule for ANKLE radiographic series in ankle injury patients	Clinical decision rule for FOOT radiographic series in ankle injury patients
Age 55 or greater	Bone tenderness (at the navicular, the cuboid, or the base of the 5th metatarsal)
Unable to bear weight (both immediately and in the ED—4 steps)	
Bone tenderness at the posterior edge or tip of either malleolus	

Importance

The Ottawa Ankle Rules study provided the evidence needed for physicians to avoid the excess use of radiography in the diagnosis and management of acute ankle injuries, thus reducing cost and radiation exposure.

Updates

- Three additional phases/studies followed the development of the Ottawa Ankle Rules (OAR).
- Phase 2 [1]: Through the study of an additional 1485 patients the rules were validated and refined to again be 100% sensitive. The rules of age 55 or greater for the ankle and the cuboid criteria for the foot proved redundant as all clinically significant fractures could be identified without them. Addition of weight bearing criteria to the foot made the rules consistent with the ankle.
- Phase 3 [2]: The OARs were implemented into clinical practice across all staff in the Ottawa Civic Hospital over a 5-month period. Compared to prior measured baseline levels, in 593 patients, adhering to the rules reduced the use of ankle radiography by 28% and foot radiographs by 14%. This led to decreased cost and patient wait times without leading to an increase in the rate of missed fractures.
- Phase 4 [3]: Widescale use of the OARs involving greater than 12,000 ankle injury patients in a variety of Canadian hospitals and community settings was feasible and successful in its primary mission regardless of physician experience. This proved the rules could be applied safely and effectively at a large scale.

Bottom Line

- The Ottawa Ankle Rules continue to serve as an accurate predictive tool for which patients with ankle injuries require x-ray to rule out fracture.

References

1. Stiell IG, Greenberg GH, McKnight D, Nair RC, McDowell I, Reardon M, Stewart JP, Maloney J. Decision rules for the use of radiography in acute ankle injuries refinement and prospective validation. JAMA. 1993;269(9):1127–32.
2. Stiell IG, McKnight D, Greenberg GH, McDowell I, Nair RC, Wells GA, Johns C, Worthington JR. Implementation of the Ottawa ankle rules. JAMA. 1994;271(11):827–32.
3. Stiell I, Well G, Laupacis A, Brison R, Verbeek R, Vandemheen K, David NC. Multicentre trial to introduce the Ottawa ankle rules for use of radiography in acute ankle injuries. BMJ. 1995;311(7005):594–7.

Chapter 49
Arthroscopic Surgery in Osteoarthritis-2002

Dimitry Belogorodsky

Background

When medical therapy fails to relieve the pain of osteoarthritis, arthroscopic lavage or debridement is often recommended. Numerous uncontrolled, retrospective case series have reported substantial pain relief after arthroscopic lavage or arthroscopic debridement for osteoarthritis of the knee [1, 2]. However, the physiological basis for the pain relief is unclear. Even with this data, there are still more than 650,000 such procedures performed each year [3] at a cost of roughly $5000.

Objective

- To evaluate the efficacy of arthroscopy for osteoarthritis of the knee using a randomized, placebo-controlled trial.

Mosley JB, O'Malley K, et al. A Controlled Trial of Arthroscopic Surgery for Osteoarthritis of the Knee. N Engl J Med 2002; 347: 81-88.
Hyperlink to PDF: https://www.nejm.org/doi/full/10.1056/NEJMoa013259

D. Belogorodsky (✉)
Jefferson Health, Abington, PA, USA
e-mail: dimitrybe@pcom.edu

J. Russell, N. S. Skolnik (eds.), *Top Articles in Primary Care*,
https://doi.org/10.1007/978-3-031-25620-2_49

Design and Methods

- Patients were recruited if they had osteoarthritis of the knee as defined by the American College of Rheumatology [4], reported at least moderate knee pain on average despite maximal medical treatment for at least 6 months, and had not undergone arthroscopy of the knee during the previous 2 years.
- 180 participants were randomly assigned into three groups: arthroscopic debridement, arthroscopic lavage alone, or the placebo procedure.
  - *Lavage*: After diagnostic arthroscopy in patients in the lavage group, the joint was lavaged with at least 10 L of fluid.
  - *Debridement*: After diagnostic arthroscopy in patients in the debridement group, the joint was lavaged with at least 10 L of fluid, rough articular cartilage was shaved, loose debris was removed, all torn or degenerated meniscal fragments were trimmed, and the remaining meniscus was smoothed to a firm and stable rim.
  - *Placebo*: To preserve blinding, a standard arthroscopic debridement procedure was simulated. Three 1-cm incisions were made in the skin. The surgeon manipulated the knee as if arthroscopy were being performed. Saline was splashed to simulate the sounds of lavage but no instrument entered the portals for arthroscopy.

Results

- At no point did either the arthroscopic debridement or arthroscopic lavage alone groups have greater pain relief than the placebo group at 1 year or at 2 years.
- There was no significant difference in arthritis pain, improvement in function, or self-reported ability to walk and bend between the placebo group and the lavage group or the debridement group at 1 or 2 years.
- Objectively measured walking and stair climbing were poorer in the debridement group than in the placebo group at 2 weeks and 1 year and showed a trend toward worse functioning at 2 years.

Importance

This study provides strong evidence that arthroscopic lavage with or without debridement is not superior to a placebo procedure in improving knee pain and self-reported function. If the efficacy of arthroscopic lavage or debridement in patients with osteoarthritis of the knee is no greater than that of placebo surgery, the billions of dollars spent on such procedures annually might be put to better use and further research.

Bottom Line

- In this controlled trial involving patients with osteoarthritis of the knee, the outcomes after arthroscopic lavage or arthroscopic debridement were no better than those after a placebo procedure.

References

1. Baumgaertner MR, Cannon WD Jr, Vittore JM, Schmidt ES, Maurer RC. Arthroscopic debridement of the arthritic knee. Clin Orthop. 1990;253:197–202.
2. Livesley PJ, Doherty M, Needoff M, Moulton A. Arthroscopic lavage of osteoarthritic knees. J Bone Joint Surg Br. 1991;73:922–26.
3. Owings MF, Kozak LJ. Ambulatory and inpatient procedures in the United States, 1996. Vital and health statistics. Series 13. No. 139. Hyattsville, MD: National Center for Health Statistics; 1998.
4. Workshop on etiopathogenesis of osteoarthritis. J Rheumatol. 1986;13:1126–60.

Chapter 50
Exercise Prescriptions-2011

Bridget Smith

Background

In 1998 the American College of Sports Medicine (ACSM) published a Position Statement which gave recommendations for the quantity and quality of exercise for healthy adult individuals [1]. The guidelines were revisited in this 2011 paper, which provided updates on how much and what type of exercise as well as which individuals should participate.

Objective

- Provide evidence-based data to guide professionals on exercise prescription in healthy adults (those without chronic disease or disability whose goal is simply to improve physical fitness and health).
- Describe the quantity and quality of exercise necessary to see benefits in physical fitness and health.

Garber, C. E., Blissmer, B., Deschenes, M. R., Franklin, B. A., Lamonte, M. J., Lee, I.-M., Nieman, D. C., & Swain, D. P. (2011). Quantity and quality of exercise for developing and maintaining cardiorespiratory, musculoskeletal, and Neuromotor fitness in apparently healthy adults. Official Journal of the American College of Sports Medicine, 43(7), 1334–1359.
Hyperlink to PDF: https://pubmed.ncbi.nlm.nih.gov/21694556/

B. Smith (✉)
Jefferson Health, Abington, PA, USA
e-mail: bridget.smith2@jefferson.edu

J. Russell, N. S. Skolnik (eds.), *Top Articles in Primary Care*,
https://doi.org/10.1007/978-3-031-25620-2_50

Design and Methods

- Bibliographic search via usual computer search engines.
- Interpretation of epidemiological studies, randomized and nonrandomized clinical trials, meta-analyses, evidence-based guidelines, consensus statements, and scientific reviews.
- All references were published from 1998 to 2010.

Results

- The ACSM recommends one of the following:
  - At least 30 min of moderate-intensity cardiovascular exercise, which is 65% of maximal oxygen uptake (VO2 max), for at least 5 days per week

    (or a total of at least 150 min of moderate-intensity cardiovascular exercise per week).
  - At least 20 min of vigorous-intensity exercise, which is 80% of maximal oxygen uptake (VO2 max), for at least 3 days per week

    (or a total of at least 75 min of vigorous-intensity cardiovascular exercise per week).
  - A combination of moderate-intensity and vigorous-intensity cardiovascular exercise for at least 500–1000 MET minutes per week.

The ACMS recommends resistance training for each of the major muscle groups for 2–3 days per week in addition to neuromotor exercise and flexibility exercises.

Research shows an amount of exercise that does not meet these recommendations still will have benefit for overall health.

More data is needed on the use of interval training, but research has shown the volume of exercise is most important. Even short bursts of exercise (10 min at a time) can have benefits, especially if there are multiple bursts throughout the day.

- The goal of 10,000 steps per day is commonly sought after, but research shows there is a benefit of simply increasing an individual's daily steps by 2000.
- Some benefits of exercise listed are a decrease in all-cause mortality and CVD mortality, improvement in glucose utilization, and improved VO2 max.
- These benefits tend to go hand in hand with the level of physical activity one achieves. Healthy middle-aged and older adults with greater cardiorespiratory fitness decrease their risk of all-cause mortality and CVD-related morbidity and mortality.
- Persons with pre-existing conditions also benefit by increasing their cardiorespiratory fitness and thus experience fewer clinical events.

- Resistance training offers benefits of improving biomarkers such as body composition, blood glucose levels, insulin sensitivity, blood pressure in persons with elevated blood pressure, and these may all help treat or prevent "metabolic syndrome" [2].
- Neuromotor exercise training (e.g., yoga, tai chi) improves motor skills such as balance, coordination, gait, agility, and proprioception.

Importance

Many patients are trying to improve their overall health, and exercise is often thought of as an important component of health. While it is common knowledge that exercise has benefits, it is important to have the data that supports this widely known theory. The data summarized in this article supports the notion that the quantity and quality of exercise impacts the benefit of exercise. It provided guidelines for healthy patients who inquire about how much and what kind of exercise they should be doing.

Updates

- The ACSM has not released an updated version of this Position Statement since 2011.
- The increase in data collection from activity trackers might lead to updated recommendations, especially given the ability to track volume of exercise, steps and distance traveled, and health measures, such as heart rate.

Bottom Line

- When it comes to physical activity, "some is good; more is better."

References

1. American College of Sports Medicine Position Stand. The recommended quantity and quality of exercise for developing and maintaining cardiorespiratory and muscular fitness, and flexibility in healthy adults. Med Sci Sports Exerc. 1998;30(6):975–91. https://doi.org/10.1097/00005768-199806000-00032.
2. Malik S, Wong ND, Franklin SS, et al. Impact of the metabolic syndrome on mortality from coronary heart disease, cardiovascular disease, and all causes in United States adults. Circulation. 2004;110(10):1245–50.

Chapter 51
Early Exercise in Concussions-2019

Kevin Franco

Background

Sports-related concussions (SRC) are a common health issue and have no proven solution [1]. Until now, studies have shown that an excessive amount of exercise in early SRC recovery worsens SRC symptoms [2]. Therefore, the standard for recovery has been a "rest-is-best" mentality [3]. With this approach up to 30% of SRC patients continue to have symptoms 1 month from injury [4]. Recent studies in pediatric patients have shown a reduction in recovery time with "moderate levels of physical activity within 7 days" from the time of injury. It is important to evaluate the benefits of sub-symptomatic level exercise in order to find methods to reduce recovery time.

Objective

- To evaluate the efficacy of sub-symptomatic aerobic exercise in adolescents early in their recovery from SRC.

Leddy JJ, Haider MN, Ellis MJ, et al. Early Subthreshold Aerobic Exercise for Sport-Related Concussion: A Randomized Clinical Trial. JAMA Pediatr. 2019;173(4):319–325. doi:10.1001/jamapediatrics.2018.4397.
Hyperlink to PDF: https://jamanetwork.com/journals/jamapediatrics/fullarticle/2723523

K. Franco (✉)
Jefferson Health, Abington, PA, USA
e-mail: Kevin.franco@jefferson.edu

J. Russell, N. S. Skolnik (eds.), *Top Articles in Primary Care*,
https://doi.org/10.1007/978-3-031-25620-2_51

Design and Methods

- A parallel randomized clinical trial (RCT) testing for symptomless exercise treatment vs a placebo group using stretching exercises in their acute recovery.
- Participants were athletes between the ages of 13 and 18 years. Their SRC was diagnosed using the International Concussion in Sport Group Criteria. Their exercise tolerance was assessed using the Buffalo Concussion Treadmill Test. They were followed weekly for 30 days.
  - No interventions were done within 48 h post-concussion.
  - The experimental group, consisting of 52 participants, exercised each day either walking, jogging, riding a stationary bike, or on a treadmill. Participants' heart rates were monitored and kept below 80% the heart rate that caused symptoms during their first visit. Their HR threshold was adjusted at their weekly clinic visit [5].
  - The control group, consisting of 51 participants, was given light daily stretching exercises.
- Both groups reported symptoms daily between the hours of seven and ten o'clock PM.
- The main measured outcome was days to recovery from date of injury.
  - Recovery meant was defined by participants showed resolution of symptoms and were being able to exercise without worsening return of symptoms.
- The secondary measurement of the study looked at participants whose recovery took longer than 30 days.
- The Mann-Whitney test was used to analyze the main outcome measure or days to recovery. For the secondary outcome of participants who had delayed recovery a test of proportions was used should this be defined?

Results

- Of 165 individuals who met inclusion criteria, 52 individuals were excluded due to not wanting to participate, exercise intolerance, or dropping out. Another 10 were removed from the study due to poor compliance, concurrent illness during the study period, or failure to return to study.
- The experimental group recovered in a median of 13 days and the control group recovered in 17 days.
- The logistic parametric survival model showed that the exercise group recovered faster than the stretching group with a p-value of 0.005 and a z score of 2.82.

Importance

Sports-related concussions are a significant medical issue and are especially relevant in younger age athletes. Younger populations have the risk of missing school, after school curricular activities and their sporting events due to concussions. Minimizing the length of recovery is important to prevent this time lost and promote a healthy return to play. In this study we see the benefits of early sub-symptomatic exercise in young athletes.

Bottom Line

- Sub-symptomatic aerobic exercise in the acute phase of recovery improves recovery times in adolescents with SRC.

References

1. Laker SR. Epidemiology of concussion and mild traumatic brain injury. PM R. 2011;3(10 suppl 2):S354–8. https://doi.org/10.1016/j.pmrj.2011.07.017.
2. Kozlowski KF, Graham J, Leddy JJ, Devinney-Boymel L, Willer BS. Exercise intolerance in individuals with postconcussion syndrome. J Athl Train. 2013;48(5):627–35. https://doi.org/10.4085/1062-6050-48.5.02.
3. McCrory P, Meeuwisse W, Aubry M, et al. Consensus statement on concussion in sport—the 4th International Conference on Concussion in Sport held in Zurich, November 2012. Clin J Sport Med. 2013;23(2):89–117. https://doi.org/10.1097/JSM.0b013e31828b67cf.
4. Zemek R, Barrowman N, Freedman SB, et al. Clinical risk score for persistent postconcussion symptoms among children with acute concussion in the ED. JAMA. 2016;315(10):1014–25. https://doi.org/10.1001/jama.2016.1203.
5. Leddy JJ, Willer B. Use of graded exercise testing in concussion and return-to-activity management. Curr Sports Med Rep. 2013;12(6):370–6. https://doi.org/10.1249/JSR.0000000000000008.

Part X
Other Areas of Medicine

Susan Kuchera Fidler

Chapter 52
The Framework for Medical Records-1968

Susan Kuchera Fidler

Background

Larry Weed, MD (1923–2017), has long been credited as the father of the modern medical record. In 1968 he outlined the chaos that surrounded existing medical record keeping. At that time, there was no recommended structure for medical documentation leaving each clinician to document however they deemed most appropriate. As one can imagine, this often led to errors, incomplete or duplicative work-ups, and misdiagnoses. Medical records failed to reflect the rigors of the scientific method, lacking in organization, data analysis, and a complete list of the patient's problems.

Objective

- The article clearly establishes three goals: to create a more organized medical record, discuss expanded use of "paramedical personnel," and instill a "more positive attitude about the computer in medicine."

Weed, L. L. (1968). Medical records that guide and teach. *N Engl J Med*, *278*(11), 593-600. https://books.google.com/books?hl=en&lr=&id=Ao-ZBQAAQBAJ&oi=fnd&pg=PA19&dq=medical+records+that+guide+and+teach+pdf&ots=k-tRlWcjcy&sig=AutPp839PRZtkzFha-pDdbzCZpo#v=onepage&q=medical%20records%20that%20guide%20and%20teach%20pdf&f=false

---

S. K. Fidler (✉)
Jefferson Health, Abington, PA, USA

J. Russell, N. S. Skolnik (eds.), *Top Articles in Primary Care*,
https://doi.org/10.1007/978-3-031-25620-2_52

Summary

- Weed is critical of the extreme variability among clinicians in the initial phase of patient evaluation.
  - While completeness is expected, what that means is highly variable between clinicians.
  - He advocates that every patient should have a minimum standard set of intake interview questions by a trained interviewer, all documented electronically.
  - Paramedical personnel are integral to this step allowing the attendings to have time to analyze the data and compile a structured problem list.
- Weed points out that the traditional scientific method is typically utilized for a single problem and therefore easy to follow to the complete answer. But patients present with multiple complex co-existing problems creating a challenge for organizing and interpreting data over time.
  - He proposes utilizing a dynamic but complete list of all the patient's problems, whether differentiated or undifferentiated, and organizing the data within each numbered problem.
  - Not only are acute hospital problems, formal diagnoses, and undifferentiated symptoms represented but also the patient's relevant biopsychosocial characteristics such as smoking and home stress, as well as needed preventive screenings.
- The problem list carries with a patient through the life of their medical care and in turn improves continuity of care.
- Weed states "the patient chooses the problem and initiates the encounter; the physician must react" emphasizing the patient-centeredness of problem-oriented charting.

Importance

This article became the framework for the modern-day medical record including SOAP (subjective/objective/assessment/plan) notes, the problem list, and Problem Oriented Medical Records. It is also the first time there was an argument to move medical records to computerized systems. For most of us, it is impossible to imagine caring for patients without a framework to organize complex complaints and analyze how the data we collect informs the decision we make in patient care. In the time before Dr. Weed changed the way we document, a physician may have to read through mountains of notes, assembled in a haphazard way, to start to conceptualize each patient's story. Now, with a well-kept medical record, a whole patient's health history is organized and available for their clinician team over years of medical care.

Further, Weed appreciated the importance of continuity of care, preventive care, and the way that social factors that are inextricably linked to a patient's medical journey. His transition to problem-oriented charting allows for the whole person care that primary care physicians strive to attain today.

Updates

In the over 50 years since Weed described his model for medical record, the evolution of computer-based charting as standard of care has been slow and painful. Weed describes the importance of "thoroughness, retrievability, efficiency and economy" as hallmarks to this documentation model which most practicing clinicians would argue is nowhere near the experience of current-day Electronic Medical Records (EMRs) [1].

Weed was not only passionate about the organization of data into the medical record but envisioned a time when that structured data could be aggregated to use large amounts of data to improve the care of the individual patient through "Problem-Knowledge Couplers" [2]. Utilizing all the structured data input into an EMR, individual patients and clinicians can benefit from the data obtained from other similar patients. The hope is this scientific method combined with the power of the data amassed from many patients would eliminate any cognitive failings of any individual clinician and improve critical thinking abilities. This process laid the groundwork for the emergence of real-world evidence inquiry, an important area of current research [3].

Bottom Line

In 1968 Larry Weed proposed a medical record structure that took indiscriminate methods of documenting complex patient data and converted them to be accountable to the rigors of the scientific method by using a problem-oriented list and structured notes to reflect all data in an organized fashion and improve patient outcomes and continuity or care. The medical record with its problem list and SOAP notes that we take for granted today owes its origin to Larry Weed.

References

1. Martin SA, Sinsky CA. The map is not the territory: medical records and 21st century practice. Lancet. 2016;388(10055):2053–6.
2. Jacobs L. Interview with Lawrence Weed, MD- The father of the problem-oriented medical record looks ahead. Perm J. 2009;13(3):84–9. https://doi.org/10.7812/TPP/09-068.
3. Blonde L, Khunti K, Harris SB, Meizinger C, Skolnik NS. Interpretation and impact of real-world clinical data for the practicing clinician. Adv Ther. 2018;35(11):1763–74. https://doi.org/10.1007/s12325-018-0805-y.

Chapter 53
Establishing a Biopsychosocial Framework for Medicine-1977

Sophie K. Oh

Background

In 1977, Engel proposed a biopsychosocial model of medicine, at a time when the prevailing biomedical model appeared to be failing both patients and physicians. As a psychiatrist, he wrote at a time when psychiatry was pulled into two directions: attempting to fully accept the biomedical model in order to be taken seriously as part of the medical profession vs becoming a field distinct from the rest of medicine.

Objective

- The author advocates for all fields of medicine to embrace a biopsychosocial model of medicine which in addition to incorporating physiology includes within its framework the "social, psychological, and behavioral dimensions of illness."

Engel G. L. (1977). The need for a new medical model: a challenge for biomedicine. *Science (New York, N.Y.)*, *196*(4286), 129–136. https://www.science.org/doi/pdf/10.1126/science.847460?casa_token=dABwnzJNO_UAAAAA:0LQDNolRI_o-eRTCLPRurlqVXfcH-m8owEgcM7P_PA34oIeLti2tZun0YHy6LIQCNJGQOw0T3VslTP8

S. K. Oh (✉)
Jefferson Health, Abington, PA, USA

J. Russell, N. S. Skolnik (eds.), *Top Articles in Primary Care*, https://doi.org/10.1007/978-3-031-25620-2_53

Summary

- According to Engel, the biomedical model is
  - reductionist, in that it seeks to reduce a disease state to its biochemical markers, and
  - dualist, in that it separates somatic diseases from mental or social "problems of living," and
  - a cultural view of disease just like any other, although we tend to think about it as "truth" because it has become dogma.
- He proposes that instead of psychiatry adopting a flawed medical model, all of medicine should move towards a biopsychosocial perspective. He argues the medical model is flawed because it:
  - ignores the psychological, social, and cultural forces that cause disparities in clinical outcomes, and
  - limits treatments to therapeutics that address the biochemical deficiencies of a disease.
- The advantages of a biopsychosocial model, Engel posits, are that it
  - allows the physician to treat all people who come through her door with a problem, whether with medical treatments recommended in a way that the patient will appreciate or via referrals to other professionals, and
  - increases accuracy of diagnosis, because a physician trained in social and psychological factors is better able to listen to a patient's words and translate them into a useful framework, ultimately leading to better treatment outcomes.
- We can understand the limits of the medical model and the benefits of the biopsychosocial model with Engel's discussion of diabetes, schizophrenia, and grief, all of which have biochemical markers but whose manifestations vary greatly between patients based on social, psychological, and cultural factors.

Importance

Published in Science, a high-impact general journal not limited to medicine, Engel champions a new-at-the-time model of medicine that remains relevant. To a physician reading in 2022, some arguments in this paper seem self-evident. For example, the modern reader would take as axiomatic the statement that a patient's experience of diabetes depends not only on her lab results but also on her view of the disease and her ability to partner with her physician to find a medication regimen and lifestyle that works for her. Today's physician is well aware that his rapport with the patient—his role as "educator and psychotherapist"—influences patient outcomes [1].

These ideas were new at the time and remain important today. The article has been cited more in the past decade than in the decade after it was written. Understanding the origins of our current medical model can lead us to question parts of our healthcare system and begin to address issues that often drive patients away from traditional care, make them skeptical of evidence-based medicine, and perhaps most importantly, allow us to understand and address disparities in healthcare. Despite our lip service to the importance of social and psychological competence, we often continue to fail those whose needs are greatest and whose experience of disease does not line up with our expectations for their illness [2].

The rise of family medicine as a specialty coincided with the rise in interest in adding social and psychological dimensions to medicine, and Engel's biopsychosocial model gave a framework for this emerging specialty. Family medicine would eventually become the largest contributor to the primary care physician workforce, constituting 40% of all primary care physicians, followed by general internists and general pediatricians [3].

Updates

- The biopsychosocial model has been embraced by medical schools, emphasizing the importance of social factors in the origin and treatment of disease. It also gives us a lens through which to look at disparities of care, a critical issue for our society at the current time.
- Another current extension of George Engel's biopsychosocial model is that medical schools often now incorporate arts and humanities into curriculum with the aim of teaching students to understand the patient experience in a social context [3].
- Living up to the ideals of Engel's model remains a challenge to this day. Patients still see many doctors as overly "technological," over-ordering tests rather than truly hearing their concerns and goals.

Bottom Line

- Embracing a biopsychosocial model of medicine allows us to better understand the origin of our patients' illness, allows them to feel better appreciated, and facilitates using shared decision making to arrive at the most appropriate treatment for patients that has the greatest chance of high adherence and success.

References

1. McInerney SJ. Introducing the biopsychosocial model for good medicine and good doctors. BMJ. https://www.bmj.com/rapid-response/2011/10/29/introducing-biopsychosocial-model-good-medicine-and-good-doctors. Published June 29, 2002. Accessed 9 Apr 2022.
2. Fava GA, Sonino N. From the lesson of George Engel to current knowledge: the biopsychosocial model 40 years later. Psychother Psychosom. 2017;86(5):257–9. https://doi.org/10.1159/000478808.
3. Bazemore A, Wilkinson E, Petterson. Proportional erosion of the primary care physician workforce has continued since 2010. Am Fam Physician. 2019;100(4):211–2.

Chapter 54
Alpha Blockers and Finasteride for BPH-1996

Kevin Franco

Background

Benign Prostatic Hyperplasia (BPH) presents itself in patients as "obstructive urinary symptoms, urinary retention, urinary tract infection and hematuria" [1]. Until the early 1990s, BPH had been treated with observation or removal of prostate. In 1990 an article was published that established the efficacy of tamsulosin, and soon after other articles were published showing the efficacy of other alpha-blockers [2, 3]. In 1992 an article published in the *New England Journal of Medicine* reported the efficacy of finasteride, a 5α-reductase inhibitor [4]. This study compared terazosin, finasteride, or both to placebo.

Terazosin is a α_1-adrenergic antagonist that works by inhibiting adrenaline's effect on $\alpha -1$ adrenergic receptors, which then cause the smooth muscle in the prostate to relax. Finasteride is a 5α-reductase inhibitor that works by decreasing DHT levels in the body, which will then decrease prostate size.

Lepor, H., Williford, W. O., Barry, M. J., Brawer, M. K., Dixon, C. M., Gormley, G., Haakenson, C., Machi, M., Narayan, P., and Padley, R. J. (1996). The efficacy of terazosin, finasteride, or both in benign prostatic hyperplasia. New England Journal of Medicine, 335(8), 533–540. https://www.nejm.org/doi/full/10.1056/nejm199608223350801#article_citing_articles.

K. Franco (✉)
Jefferson Health, Abington, PA, USA

J. Russell, N. S. Skolnik (eds.), *Top Articles in Primary Care*,
https://doi.org/10.1007/978-3-031-25620-2_54

Objective

- Study the efficacy and safety of terazosin, finasteride, and the combination of terazosin and finasteride compared to placebo in males with BPH.

Design and Methods

- A double-blind, placebo-controlled study including men between the ages of 45 and 80 years of age.
- Participants were given placebo for a 4-week single blind run-in period.
- Symptoms were scored using the American Urological Association Symptom Index, where 1–7 is mild, 8–19 is moderate, and 20–35 is severe.
- In addition to symptoms, other measures included patients' peak urinary flow rates, PSA, and post-void residual volumes.
- Inclusion criteria required a symptom score of 8 and above, residual volume below 300 mL, and mean urinary flow rate between 4 and 15 mL/s. Prostate size was measured but not used in inclusion criteria.
- After the 4-week placebo run-in, patients were randomized to terazosin, finasteride, a combination of terazosin and finasteride, or placebo.
- Symptom scores, peak urinary flow rates, and residual post-void volumes were retested 10 times over 1 year and compared to their baseline scores.

Results

- 1229 of the original 1686 participants met criteria and were included in this study.
- Symptomatic scores were significantly decreased in the terazosin and combination groups.
- Although changes were seen in the placebo and finasteride group, there was no significant difference from baseline for finasteride alone.
- Urinary flow rates and symptoms scores were significantly improved in terazosin and combination groups vs. placebo. Finasteride alone did not significantly differ in effect on urinary flow rate from placebo.
- Patients in the terazosin group and combination group had significantly more dizziness and required more dose reductions than placebo.
- Patients in the finasteride and combinations groups had the most impotence while the combination group had significantly more ejaculatory abnormalities.
- Prostatic volume changes were significantly decreased in the combination and finasteride vs. terazosin and placebo group.

Importance

Before this article in 1996, there were no studies comparing the use of finasteride, terazosin, and both in combination for the treatment of BPH. Previous studies had shown the safety and efficacy of both finasteride and terazosin individually. This study's findings were similar to previous study results with regard to the effect of terazosin but showed finasteride to have no advantage over the course of the year in symptomatic improvement compared to placebo. In previous studies the outcome for finasteride versus placebo group was statistically significant but was small. The paper hypothesizes that prior studies of finasteride enrolled patients with much larger prostates therefore resulting in increased efficacy of finasteride. The effect from the combination of terazosin and finasteride on symptoms and flow rate at 1 year was not statistically greater than terazosin alone.

Bottom Line

- Terazosin was shown to be significantly better than finasteride and placebo at symptomatic reduction and improved urinary flow in BPH patients.
- Finasteride alone showed no benefit on symptoms and flow rate at 1 year compared to placebo.
- The addition of finasteride to terazosin showed no more improvement compared to terazosin alone on symptoms and flow rate at 1 year.
- This study advanced our understanding of the diverse underlying pathophysiology of BPH and its relation to treatment efficacy. This led to the modern approach to therapy, as articulated in the accompanying editorial to this paper, "If a man with such symptoms does not have an enlarged prostate gland on digital rectal examination, he should be treated with an α1-adrenergic–antagonist drug. Conversely, if the prostate gland is enlarged, as it is in nearly a quarter of men 60–69 years of age, then treatment with either finasteride or an α1-adrenergic antagonist is a reasonable option" [5].
- This led to the current approach to treatment which recommend quantifying symptoms and examining the prostate. Alpha-blockers are a good first choice for all men with symptoms. If someone has an enlarged prostate, defined as >30 g on rectal exam or imaging or reflected by a prostate-specific antigen (PSA) level > 1.5 ng/dL, then a 5-alpha reductase inhibitor, such as finasteride or dutasteride, either alone or in combination with an alpha-blocker is recommended [6, 7].

References

1. Madsen FA, Bruskewitz RC. Clinical manifestations of benign prostatic hyperplasia. Urol Clin North Am. 1995;22(2):291–8.
2. Kawabe K, Ueno A, Takimoto Y, Aso Y, Kato H. Use of alpha$_1$-blocker, YM617, in the treatment of benign prostatic hypertrophy. J Urol. 1990;144:908–11.
3. Lepor H, Auerbach S, Puras-Baez A, et al. A randomized, placebo-controlled multicenter study of the efficacy and safety of terazosin in the treatment of benign prostatic hyperplasia. J Urol. 1992;148:1467–74.
4. Gormley GJ, Stoner E, Bruskewitz RC, et al. The effect of finasteride in men with benign prostatic hyperplasia. N Engl J Med. 1992;327:1185–91.
5. Walsh PC. Treatment of benign prostatic hyperplasia. N Engl J Med. 1996;335:586–7.
6. Skolnik NS. Managing the lower urinary tract symptoms of BPH: new guidance. Medscape. 2022. https://www.medscape.com/viewarticle/965388.
7. Management of benign prostatic hyperplasia/lower urinary tract symptoms: AUA guideline. 2021. https://www.auanet.org/guidelines/guidelines/benign-prostatic-hyperplasia-(bph)-guideline.

Chapter 55
Sildenafil for Erectile Dysfunction-1998

Karen Lazarus

Background

Erectile Dysfunction (ED) is the consistent or recurrent inability to acquire or sustain an erection of sufficient rigidity and duration for sexual intercourse [1]. It is the most common form of male sexual dysfunction, affecting more than 18 million men aged 20 or older in the USA [2]. This disorder is associated with age with estimated prevalence rates of 39% among men 40 years old and 67% among those 70 years old [3]. This study was the first to demonstrate that sildenafil, a phosphodiesterase type 5 (PDE-5) inhibitor, was an effective treatment for men with ED when there were no other oral therapies available. Interestingly, PDE-5 inhibitors were originally developed to treat angina pectoris. However, the requirement for frequent dosing and interactions with nitrates made this problematic. During clinical trials, volunteers reported penile erections as a side effect and clinical trials investigating the use of PDE-5 inhibitors for ED began in 1993 [4].

Goldstein, I., Lue, T. F., Padma-Nathan, H., Rosen, R. C., Steers, W. D., and Wicker, P. A. (1998). Oral sildenafil in the treatment of erectile dysfunction. Sildenafil Study Group. The New England Journal of Medicine, 338(20), 1397–1404.
Hyperlink to PDF: https://www.nejm.org/doi/pdf/10.1056/NEJM199805143382001?articleTools=true.

K. Lazarus (✉)
Jefferson Health, Abington, PA, USA

J. Russell, N. S. Skolnik (eds.), *Top Articles in Primary Care*,
https://doi.org/10.1007/978-3-031-25620-2_55

Objective

- To evaluate the efficacy, safety, and dose–response of sildenafil as treatment for ED.

Design and Methods

- Two sequential studies with 861 participants aged 18 years or older with a clinical diagnosis of ED were done to assess (1) the efficacy and safety of the medication and (2) to assess the dose–response relationship.
  - The first study was a 24-week *dose–response study* where 532 men were treated with oral sildenafil (25, 50, or 100 mg) or placebo 1 h before sexual activity.
  - The second study was a 12-week flexible *dose-escalation study* where 329 different men were treated with sildenafil or placebo 1 h before sexual activity. The dose was escalated to 100 mg based on efficacy and tolerance.

    After this dose-escalation study, the 225 men who had no serious side effects entered a 32-week open label extension study.

Efficacy was assessed via International Index of Erectile Function (a self-report instrument to evaluate male sexual function), patient log, and a global efficacy question.

- Mean domain scores from the International Index of Erectile Function were analyzed with an analysis-of-covariance model that was fitted for each question.
- From the event log, the mean numbers of substantial erections (in the dose–response study) or the percentage of attempts at sexual intercourse that were successful (in the dose-escalation study) was calculated via analysis of covariance (dose–response study) or a chi-square test (dose-escalation study).
- The answers of each treatment group to the global efficacy question (yes or no) were analyzed with the use of logistic regression analysis.
- Adjustments were made for the following covariates: patient age, smoking, and duration and cause of ED.

Results

- In the dose–response study, increasing doses of sildenafil were significantly associated with improved erectile function.
- In the dose-escalation study, the men receiving sildenafil were three times as likely to have successful intercourse compared to those receiving placebo.

- The mean numbers of successful attempts per month were nearly four times greater for the men receiving sildenafil than for those receiving placebo.
- Headache, flushing, and dyspepsia were the most common adverse effects, occurring in 6–18% of the men. Sildenafil has modest vasodilator properties but no effect on heart rate. No man had priapism after sildenafil treatment.

Importance

Until the publication of this article in 1998, there were no oral medications for the treatment of ED. Sildenafil (which was marketed by the pharmaceutical company Pfizer as Viagra) was the first FDA-approved oral medication for this purpose. Administration of sildenafil is discrete and simple compared to other treatment options available at the time, such as corpus cavernosum injections, transurethral drug delivery, vacuum pressure devices, and prosthesis implantation [5]. Today, PDE-5 inhibitors are first-line treatment for ED. These include sildenafil, vardenafil, tadalafil, and avanafil [6]. All PDE-5 inhibitors have FDA approval for the treatment of ED. Sildenafil is also approved for the treatment of pulmonary hypertension. Tadalafil is approved for ED, pulmonary hypertension, and benign prostatic hyperplasia (BPH) with or without ED.

Bottom Line

- Sildenafil is a PDE-5 inhibitor that was the first FDA-approved oral medication to treat ED. This publication, which outlined two sequential studies, consisted of 861 participants aged 18 years or older with a clinical diagnosis of ED showed that the medication was effective, safe, and that higher doses improved erections. Headache, flushing, and dyspepsia were the most common symptoms. PDE-5 inhibitors are contraindicated in men taking nitrates and should be used cautiously in men receiving an alpha-adrenergic blocker due to increased risk of hypotension [7].

References

1. National Institutes of Health. NIH consensus conference. Impotence. NIH consensus development panel on impotence. JAMA. 1993;270:83–90.
2. Selvin E, Burnett AL, Platz EA. Prevalence and risk factors for erectile dysfunction in the US. Am J Med. 2007;120(2):151–7.
3. Feldman HA, et al. Impotence and its medical and psychosocial correlates: results of the Massachusetts male aging study. J Urol. 1994;151(1):54–61.

4. Ghofrani HA, et al. Sildenafil: from angina to erectile dysfunction to pulmonary hypertension and beyond. Nat Rev Drug Discov. 2006;5(8):689–702.
5. Gurtner K, et al. Erectile dysfunction: a review of historical treatments with a focus on the development of the inflatable penile prosthesis. Am J Mens Health. 2017;11(3):479–86.
6. Tsertsvadze A, et al. Oral phosphodiesterase-5 inhibitors and hormonal treatments for erectile dysfunction: a systematic review and meta-analysis. Ann Intern Med. 2009;151(9):650.
7. Full prescribing information: viagra (sildenafil citrate) tablets for oral use. 2017. http://labeling.pfizer.com/ShowLabeling.aspx?format=PDF&id=652.

Chapter 56
A Randomized Trial Comparing Conventional and Endovascular Repair of Abdominal Aortic Aneurysms-2008

Marissa Norden

Background

Patients with abdominal aortic aneurysms will require close monitoring and should undergo elective repair when the aneurysm reaches a diameter of 5–5.5 cm. Diameter of aneurysm is directly related to risk of rupture, with aneurysms >5 cm having up to a 15% rupture rate over the next year [1]. Endovascular repair was introduced in 1991 as an alternative to open repair. Early benefits were seen but the procedure needed to be compared to the standard of care in a randomized controlled trial in order to know that the benefits seen were not just from patient selection [2]. This study looked to compare and contrast outcomes in patients who received endovascular repair in comparison to open repair in patients with similar baseline characteristics.

Objective

- To compare the perioperative mortality and complications over 30 days between endovascular and open approaches of repair of abdominal aortic aneurysms.

Prinssen, M, Verhoeven, E (et al.). (2004). A Randomized Trial Comparing Conventional and Endovascular Abdominal Aortic Aneurysm Repair. New England Journal of Medicine, 351(16), 1607–1618.
https://www.nejm.org/doi/full/10.1056/NEJMoa042002.

M. Norden (✉)
Jefferson Health, Abington, PA, USA
e-mail: Marissa.Norden@jefferson.edu

J. Russell, N. S. Skolnik (eds.), *Top Articles in Primary Care*,
https://doi.org/10.1007/978-3-031-25620-2_56

Design and Methods

- Patients from 28 surgical centers were randomly assigned to endovascular or open repair.
- Certain exclusions included patients with inflammatory aneurysms, connective tissue disease, organ transplant recipients, patients with life expectancy less than 2 years, or need for urgent repair of aneurysm.
- Surgical teams needed to have completed at least 5 previous endovascular repairs.
- Randomization of patients ensured that they had similar baseline characteristics.
- There were originally 345 patients, and 174 were assigned to open repair and 171 were assigned to endovascular repair. Given the need for a few conversions and crossovers of procedure type, open repair was completed in 173 patients and endovascular repair was completed in 171 patients.

Results

- General anesthesia was required in 98% of open cases and 54.9% of endovascular cases.
- Mortality during surgery: 4.6% of open cases, 1.2% of endovascular cases; Risk ratio of 3.9 and *p*-value of 0.1.
- Mortality or severe complications within 30 days occurred in 9.8% of open cases and 4.7% of endovascular cases, with a *p*-value of 0.1.
- Mortality or moderate or severe complications within 30 days occurred in 23% of open cases and 18% endovascular cases with a *p*-value 0.23. Moderate complications often included local complications such as graft leaks, infections, or obstructions.
- Systemic complications occurred in 26.4% of open cases, and 11.7% of endovascular with a *p*-value <001. Most commonly included cardiac or pulmonary complications.
- Local vascular complications occurred in 8.6% of open cases and in 16.4% of endovascular cases with *p*-value of 0.03. These often include hemorrhage, graft complications, and graft leaks.
- Open cases were on average longer (151 min) than endovascular cases (135 min) with a *p*-value of <001.
- There was less blood loss (354 mL) in endovascular cases in comparison to open cases (1654 mL), with less need for blood transfusion in endovascular cases. *P*-value <001.
- Shorter ICU stay in endovascular cases (16 h vs. 72 h) as well as shorter period on ventilator, and shorter hospitalizations with endovascular repair (6 vs. 13 days) *P*-value <001.

Importance

Endovascular repair appears to be better than open repair in the perioperative period and first 30 days. It was associated with decreased perioperative morality, decreased systemic complications, shorter surgery times, shorter hospital stays, and decreased blood loss. Endovascular repair did not lead to a statistically significant improvement when looking at moderate complications, as it tends to be associated with higher local complications. This is important when looking at both patient and hospital goals. However, this study is only relevant when looking at patients that would qualify for both open and endovascular repair, and many patients would not be candidates for endovascular repair. This study also only looked at patients getting an elective repair and not an urgent repair. Patients undergoing endovascular procedure need to be aware of increased risks of local complications as well.

Update

While this trial showed that endovascular repair has substantial advantages over open repair both perioperatively and in the first 30 days, it remained to be seen what the long-term outcomes would be. In longer-term follow-up of randomized trials, the early mortality benefit appears to wane over time, perhaps due to the higher re-intervention rate over time. Data on long-term follow-up is limited, with one randomized trial showing improved mortality to endovascular repair lasting for 6 months, and by 8 years a mortality benefit to open repair. An observational study with data out to 12 years showed no significant mortality difference between the two procedures [2].

Bottom Line

- Perioperative mortality and systemic complication decreased in endovascular repair of aortic aneurysms compared to open repair; endovascular repair did have higher local complications.
- Endovascular repair had a statistically significant decrease in length of surgery, need for transfusion, and decrease in surgery time, which can be beneficial for both patients and hospital systems.
- Limits to endovascular repair include cost, need for training, and many patients are not candidates for this procedure.
- In order to be considered for endovascular repair, patients need to have certain anatomic features. Patients with calcifications or tortuosity of the aorta or iliac artery are not candidates for endovascular repair.

- Endovascular repair offers clear advantages over the short term, and with the improvements in the technology, may offer advantages both short and long term, though long-term data is limited, particularly with more modern grafts.
- Decisions therefore need to be individualized based on both anatomy and shared decision making incorporating patient preferences.

References

1. Swerdlow NJ, Wu WW, Schermerhorn ML. Open and endovascular management of aortic aneurysms. Circ Res. 2019;124(4):647–61.
2. Salata K, Hussain M, Mestral C. Comparison of outcomes in elective endovascular aortic repair vs open surgical repair of abdominal aortic aneurysms. JAMA Netw Open. 2019;2(7):e196578.

Part XI
Pediatrics

John Russell

Chapter 57
Sleeping Position and SIDS-1993

Gerard Cleary and Sean Cleary

Background

The prone sleeping position has been implicated as an impetus of sudden infant death syndrome (SIDS) in several retrospective studies, though the association is poorly understood [1]. SIDS is the unexplained death of an otherwise healthy baby less than a year old and usually occurs during sleep. Data analysis from a case-control study and prospective cohort study in Tasmania, Australia, sought to identify conditions that potentiate the risk of SIDS in infants that were in the prone sleeping position. The results from this study indicate that four factors increase the risk of SIDS while prone: the use of natural fiber mattresses, swaddling, recent illness, and the use of heating in the bedroom.

Ponsonby, A.-L., Dwyer, T., Gibbons, L. E., Cochrane, J. A., & Wang, Y.-G. (1993). Factors potentiating the risk of sudden infant death syndrome associated with the prone position. New England Journal of Medicine, 329(6), 377–382. https://doi.org/10.1056/nejm199308053290601. https://www.nejm.org/doi/pdf/10.1056/NEJM199308053290601?articleTools=true.

G. Cleary (✉)
Jefferson Health, Abington, PA, USA
e-mail: Gerard.Cleary@jefferson.edu

S. Cleary
Jefferson Health, Abington, PA, USA

Philadelphia College of Osteopathic Medicine, PCOM, Philadelphia, PA, USA
e-mail: sc208239@pcom.edu

J. Russell, N. S. Skolnik (eds.), *Top Articles in Primary Care*,
https://doi.org/10.1007/978-3-031-25620-2_57

Objective

- To identify effect modifiers of the connection between prone sleeping position and sudden infant death syndrome (SIDS) by analyzing data from Tasmanian case-control and prospective cohort studies.

Design and Methods

- The case-control study analyzed in this report consisted of infants born in Tasmania, Australia. Infants in the case group were classified as having died from SIDS. For each case infant, 2 control infants were included in the study: 1 control infant was matched for age and 1 control infant was matched for age and birth weight. Reports on thermal environment at time of death were collected on scene or obtained via parental interview for some case infants. Thermal measurements for control infants were obtained at the infant's homes by a research assistant. All additional information was obtained via a comprehensive verbal questionnaire administered to case parents approximately 6 weeks after their child had died and to control parents directly after measurement of thermal environment.
- The cohort prospective study included approximately 20% of live-born infants in Tasmania who were classified as being at increased risk for SIDS between January 1988 and June 1991. Data was analyzed to identify the effect modification of the prone position to the type of mattress used.
- Statistical analysis was performed on the results from these two studies to determine variables that contribute to SIDS in the prone position.
- For the case-control study, odds ratios were calculated to assess the association between SIDS and selected variables in accordance with the infant's usual sleeping position (supine/on the side or prone). The variables included in the study were: mattress used, infant swaddling, recent illness, and room heat.
- For the cohort study, conditional logistic regression was used to assess the interaction between the usual sleeping position of the infant and the type of mattress used.

Results

- In the case-control study, risk of SIDS was significantly higher in those infants who slept prone in comparison to those who slept supine or on their sides.
- The risk of SIDS in infants sleeping in the prone position was enhanced 20-fold for those sleeping on natural-fiber mattresses. This term refers to mattresses filled with flakes of ti-tree bark or kapok fibers enclosed in a permeable cotton cover (as opposed to foam mattresses which are considered non-natural in the study). For prone sleeping infants on mattresses not filled with natural fibers (i.e., foam mattresses), the risk of SIDS was only increased threefold.
- There was a 12-fold increase in risk for SIDS in infants sleeping in the prone position that were swaddled (i.e., wrapped in any item of bedding such as a blan-

ket or sheet while asleep), compared to a threefold increase in non-swaddled prone sleepers.

- A tenfold increase in risk of SIDS was observed in prone infants that were ill with nasal congestion, cough, chest noises, fever, vomiting, or diarrhea the day of death or the day prior. Illness was not associated with a higher risk of SIDS among infants who slept supine or on their side.
- The effect of prone position on the risk of SIDS was enhanced in infants sleeping in warmer rooms (15–29 °C) than in cooler rooms (6–14 °C).

Importance

The seminal article by Ponsonby, published in 1993 evaluating sleep position and risks for sudden infant death syndrome, was not without controversy [2]. In fact, it went against the prevailing medical and cultural beliefs that children should sleep on their stomachs to prevent aspiration in the event of regurgitation. The fact that infants commonly wet burp or have recognizable reflux and the concern for aspiration and death were the prevailing beliefs for grandmothers and doctors alike to recommend prone sleeping position. With the publication of this article, the first epidemiologic study to challenge these beliefs, the American Academy of Pediatrics, the National Institute of Child Health and Development (now the Eunice Kennedy Shriver Institute of Child Health and development), and multiple other child advocacy groups initiated the "Back to Sleep" campaign. Between 1992 and 2001, the SIDS rate declined by 50%. The increase in supine positioning for sleep directly correlated with the decrease in SIDS deaths during these years [3] (see Fig. 57.1). https://www.cdc.gov/sids/data.htm#graph.

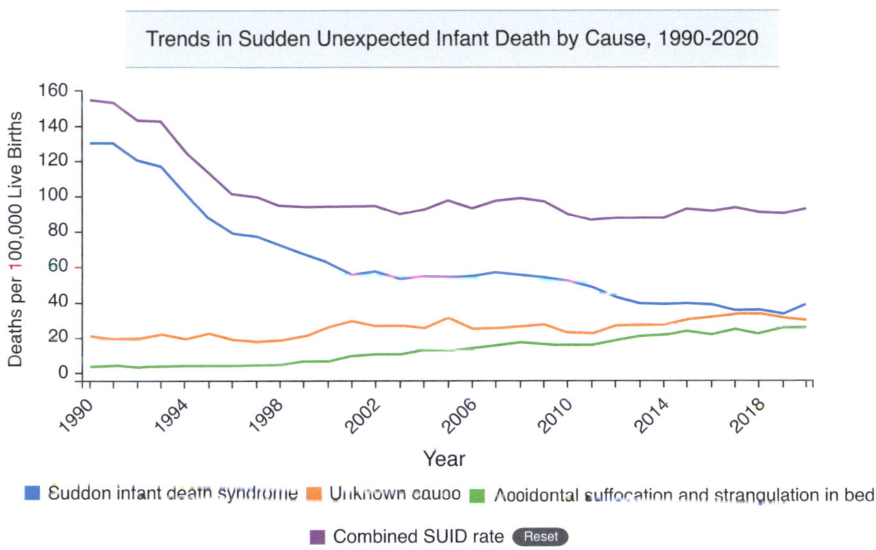

Fig. 57.1 Trends in sudden infant death [4]

While the physiologic understanding of SIDS remains unknown, the risks can be defined by several categories including a vulnerable infant who is exposed to exogenous stressors during a critical developmental period [5]. This understanding has helped medical examiners to refine the definition of SIDS and differentiate accidental suffocation and strangulation in bed [6]. Sudden unexpected infant death (SUID) is the combination of these two and has also declined in the years since the "Back to Sleep" campaign became the "Safe Sleep" campaign. Furthermore, supine positioning does not increase the risk of aspiration or choking, even in infants with gastroesophageal reflux. Multiple studies have demonstrated no change in incidence of aspiration or choking since the change to supine positioning [7, 8].

Updates

- It is also important to note that "Safe Sleep" campaign has introduced additional modification in sleeping environment, all directed toward modifying the exogenous stressors to a vulnerable child. Each has its own risk reduction ratio that further drives down the SUID rates. These include attention to sleep surfaces to include only a firm flat mattress with fitted bedding, a crib, bassinet, or portable crib that conforms to Consumer Product Safety Commission guidelines. Others include avoidance of car seats, strollers, or swings for routine sleep, encouraging breast feeding, infants sleeping in the parents' room but on a separate surface, avoid co-bedding with parents, smoking and alcohol use. Infants should never be placed on sofas or recliners for sleeping and bumpers in cribs should be avoided. Table 57.1 has OR for these behaviors and environmental factors. Finally, there is no evidence that apparent life-threatening events are precursors to SIDS. Infant home cardiorespiratory monitors should not be used as a strategy to reduce the risk of SIDS [28–30].

Table 57.1 Odds ratio for environmental or behavior modification

Environmental or behavior modification	Odds ratio	Source
Prone positioning	2.4–13.1	[9, 10]
Side positioning	2.0–2.6	[11]
Soft bedding/memory foam	5.1	[9, 12, 13]
Bed sharing	2.7–10.2	[14–16]
Room sharing	0.67–1	[14–16]
Car seats, strollers, swings	1.68–7.35	[17]
Breast feeding	0.27–0.64	[18, 19]
Smoking	1.6–4.1	[20, 21]
Pacifier use	0.14–0.62	[22–24]
Alcohol, drugs	2.3–3.6	[24]
Sharing sofas, recliners	18–66.9	[14, 15]
Overheating	1.14–2.7	[25–27]

Bottom Line

- The pathophysiology of SUID remains unclear. Multiple hypotheses include dysfunctional cardiorespiratory or arousal protective responses that are manifestations of environmental conditions, genetic maldevelopment, delay in maturation, or infectious triggers. The convergence of these factors may result in progressive hypoxemia, bradycardia, acidosis, and dismissed gasping leading to unexplained death. The triple risk model of SIDS arises from these considerations and is the fatal combination of exogenous stressors, critical developmental period, and a vulnerable infant that leads to unexpected death. Each of the "safe sleep" recommendations addresses minimizing environmental stressors and identifying and modifying conditions for the vulnerable infant. Identifying genetic [31], biochemical, and clinical markers to assess risk of SIDS is an area of ongoing research and includes evaluation of Butyrylcholinesterase as a potential biomarker [32], as well as evaluating signal to noise ratio during newborn hearing screening to proactively identify infants as increased risk [33]. These investigations are ongoing and have not yielded an actionable clinical approach to early identification of at-risk infants
- Ongoing work to narrow the ethnic and racial disparities in SIDS rates and adoption of "safe sleep" practices remains a critical component for healthcare providers and public health professionals [34, 35]
- The vigilance of parents to modify the environment for safe sleep is our best approach to SIDS prevention and started with the epidemiological studies of Ponsonby et al. in the classic article reviewed in this chapter.

References

1. Ponsonby A-L, Dwyer T, Gibbons LE, Cochrane JA, Wang Y-G. Factors potentiating the risk of sudden infant death syndrome associated with the prone position. N Engl J Med. 1993;329(6):377–82. https://doi.org/10.1056/nejm199308053290601.
2. Chole SD, Gibbons L, Dwyer T, Ponsonby A-L, Shannon DC, Li D-K, Thach BT, Kemp JS. The risk of sudden infant death. N Engl J Med. 1994;330(1):63–4. https://doi.org/10.1056/nejm199401063300113.
3. Moon RY. SIDS and other sleep-related infant deaths: evidence base for 2016 updated recommendations for a safe infant sleeping environment. Pediatrics. 2017;138(5):1213–46. https://doi.org/10.1542/9781610020862-part04-environment.
4. Centers for Disease Control and Prevention. Data and statistics for SIDS and SUID. Atlanta, GA: Centers for Disease Control and Prevention; 2022. https://www.cdc.gov/sids/data.htm. Accessed 30 Jun 2022.
5. Filiano JJ, Kinney HC. A perspective on neuropathologic findings in victims of the sudden infant death syndrome: the triple-risk model. Neonatology. 1994;65(3–4):194–7. https://doi.org/10.1159/000244052.
6. Willinger M, James LS, Catz C. Defining the sudden infant death syndrome (SIDS): deliberations of an expert panel convened by the national institute of child health and human development. Pediatr Pathol. 1991;11(5):677–84. https://doi.org/10.3109/15513819109065465.

7. Byard R, Beal S. Gastric aspiration and sleeping position in infancy and early childhood. J Paediatr Child Health. 2000;36(4):403–5. https://doi.org/10.1046/j.1440-1754.2000.00503.x.
8. Tablizo MA, Jacinto P, Parsley D, Chen ML, Ramanathan R, Keens TG. Supine sleeping position does not cause clinical aspiration in neonates in hospital newborn nurseries. Arch Pediatr Adolesc Med. 2007;161(5):507. https://doi.org/10.1001/archpedi.161.5.507.
9. Hauck FR, Herman SM, Donovan M, Iyasu S, Merrick Moore C, Donoghue E, Kirschner RH, Willinger M. Sleep environment and the risk of sudden infant death syndrome in an urban population: the Chicago infant mortality study. Pediatrics. 2003;111(Supplement_1):1207–14. https://doi.org/10.1542/peds.111.s1.1207.
10. Carpenter RG, Irgens LM, Blair PS, England PD, Fleming P, Huber J, Jorch G, Schreuder P. Sudden unexplained infant death in 20 regions in Europe: case control study. Lancet. 2004;363(9404):185–91. https://doi.org/10.1016/s0140-6736(03)15323-8.
11. Li D-K. Infant sleeping position and the risk of sudden infant death syndrome in California, 1997-2000. Am J Epidemiol. 2003;157(5):446–55. https://doi.org/10.1093/aje/kwf226.
12. Kemp JS, Livne M, White DK, Arfken CL. Softness and potential to cause rebreathing: differences in bedding used by infants at high and low risk for sudden infant death syndrome. J Pediatr. 1998;132(2):234–9. https://doi.org/10.1016/s0022-3476(98)70437-8.
13. Kemp JS, Nelson VE, Thach BT. Physical properties of bedding that may increase risk of sudden infant death syndrome in prone-sleeping infants. Pediatr Res. 1994;36:7–11. https://doi.org/10.1203/00006450-199407001-00002.
14. Blair PS, Fleming PJ, Smith IJ, Platt MW, Young J, Nadin P, Berry PJ, Golding J, Mitchell E, The CESDI SUDI Research Group. Babies sleeping with parents: case-control study of factors influencing the risk of the sudden infant death syndrome commentary: cot death—the story so far. BMJ. 1999;319(7223):1457–62. https://doi.org/10.1136/bmj.319.7223.1457.
15. Tappin D, Brooke H, Ecob R. Bedsharing and sudden infant death syndrome (SIDS) in Scotland, UK. Lancet. 2004;363(9413):994. https://doi.org/10.1016/s0140-6736(04)15806-6.
16. Carpenter R, McGarvey C, Mitchell EA, Tappin DM, Vennemann MM, Smuk M, Carpenter JR. Bed sharing when parents do not smoke: is there a risk of SIDS? An individual level analysis of five major case–control studies. BMJ Open. 2013;3(5):e002299. https://doi.org/10.1136/bmjopen-2012-002299.
17. Cote A, Bairam A, Deschenes M, Hatzakis G. Sudden infant deaths in sitting devices. Arch Dis Child. 2008;93(5):384–9. https://doi.org/10.1136/adc.2007.119180.
18. Vennemann MM, Bajanowski T, Brinkmann B, Jorch G, Yücesan K, Sauerland C, Mitchell EA. Does breastfeeding reduce the risk of sudden infant death syndrome? Pediatrics. 2009;123(3):e406–10. https://doi.org/10.1542/peds.2008-2145.
19. Hauck FR, Thompson JM, Tanabe KO, Moon RY, Vennemann MM. Breastfeeding and reduced risk of sudden infant death syndrome: a meta-analysis. Pediatrics. 2011;128(1):103–10. https://doi.org/10.1542/peds.2010-3000.
20. MacDorman MF, Cnattingius S, Hoffman HJ, Kramer MS, Haglund B. Sudden infant death syndrome and smoking in the United States and Sweden. Am J Epidemiol. 1997;146(3):249–57. https://doi.org/10.1093/oxfordjournals.aje.a009260.
21. Haglund B, Cnattingius S. Cigarette smoking as a risk factor for sudden infant death syndrome: a population-based study. Am J Public Health. 1990;80(1):29–32. https://doi.org/10.2105/ajph.80.1.29.
22. Hauck FR, Omojokun OO, Siadaty MS. Do pacifiers reduce the risk of sudden infant death syndrome? A meta-analysis. Pediatrics. 2005;116(5):e716–23. https://doi.org/10.1542/peds.2004-2631.
23. Mitchell EA, Blair PS, L'Hoir MP. Should pacifiers be recommended to prevent sudden infant death syndrome? Pediatrics. 2006;117(5):1755–8. https://doi.org/10.1542/peds.2005-1625.
24. Kandall SR, Gaines J, Habel L, Davidson G, Jessop D. Relationship of maternal substance abuse to subsequent sudden infant death syndrome in offspring. J Pediatr. 1993;123(1):120–6. https://doi.org/10.1016/s0022-3476(05)81554-9.

25. Fleming PJ, Gilbert R, Azaz Y, Berry PJ, Rudd PT, Stewart A, Hall E. Interaction between bedding and sleeping position in the sudden infant death syndrome: a population based case-control study. BMJ. 1990;301(6743):85–9. https://doi.org/10.1136/bmj.301.6743.85.
26. Fleming PJ, Blair P. Thermal environment and the risk of sudden infant death: epidemiology and developmental physiology. Ambul Child Health. 2000;6(s1):26–7. https://doi.org/10.1046/j.1467-0658.2000.00011.x.
27. Ponsonby AL, Dwyer T, Gibbons LE, Cochrane JA, Jones ME, McCall MJ. Thermal environment and sudden infant death syndrome: case-control study. BMJ. 1992;304(6822):277–82. https://doi.org/10.1136/bmj.304.6822.277.
28. Ward SL, Keens TG, Chan LS, Chipps BE, Carson SH, Deming DD, Krishna V, MacDonald HM, Martin GI, Meredith KS, Merritt TA, Nickerson BG, Stoddard RA, van der Hal AL. Sudden infant death syndrome in infants evaluated by APNEA programs in California. Pediatrics. 1986;77(4):451–8. https://doi.org/10.1542/peds.77.4.451.
29. Ramanathan R. Cardiorespiratory events recorded on home monitors comparison of healthy infants with those at increased risk for sids. JAMA. 2001;285(17):2199. https://doi.org/10.1001/jama.285.17.2199.
30. Committee on Fetus and Newborn. American Academy of Pediatrics. Apnea, sudden infant death syndrome, and home monitoring. Pediatrics. 2003;111(4):914–7. https://doi.org/10.1542/peds.111.4.914.
31. Steer J, Annavarapu S. The genetics of sudden infant death syndrome. In: Cohen MC, Scheimberg IB, Beckwith JB, Hauck F, editors. Investigation of sudden infant death syndrome; 2019. p. 159–71. https://doi.org/10.1017/9781108186001.028
32. Harrington CT, Hafid NA, Waters KA. Butyrylcholinesterase is a potential biomarker for sudden infant death syndrome. EBioMedicine. 2022;80:104041. https://doi.org/10.1016/j.ebiom.2022.104041.
33. Rubens DD, Vohr BR, Tucker R, O'Neil CA, Chung W. Newborn Oto-acoustic emission hearing screening tests. Early Hum Dev. 2008;84(4):225–9. https://doi.org/10.1016/j.earlhumdev.2007.06.001.
34. Oden RP, Joyner BL, Ajao TI, Moon RY. Factors influencing African American mothers' decisions about sleep position: a qualitative study. J Natl Med Assoc. 2010;102(10):870–80. https://doi.org/10.1016/s0027-9684(15)30705-7.
35. Colson ER, McCabe LK, Fox K, Levenson S, Colton T, Lister G, Corwin MJ. Barriers to following the back-to-sleep recommendations: insights from focus groups with inner-city caregivers. Ambul Pediatr. 2005;5(6):349–54. https://doi.org/10.1367/a04-220r1.1.

Chapter 58
MMR and Autism 1998

Christian Iversen

Summary of Original Paper

- Reported and actual methods/results were discrepant, see "Updates" for additional information. *The publication was eventually retracted for numerous ethical and scientific issues.*
- The authors suggested they were investigating potential causes for a regressive developmental disorder in children with chronic enterocolitis. They enrolled 12 children (mean age 6; 11 males, 1 female) who were referred to gastroenterology for a combination of intestinal symptoms (diarrhea, abdominal pain, bloating, and food intolerance) and developmental regression.
- Investigators collected developmental and exposure history and performed psychiatric assessments. Patients were further examined with ileocolonoscopy with biopsies, MRI, EEG, lumbar puncture, and barium follow-through. Laboratory studies were performed to test for known neurodegenerative or infectious conditions.
- Children were suggested to be developmentally normal prior to displaying developmental regression. No abnormalities were identified on neurologic examination, MRI, EEG, or lumbar puncture. Fragile X testing was negative. Infectious studies were negative.

Wakefield AJ, Murch SH, Anthony A, Linnell J, Casson DM, Malik M, Berelowitz M, Dhillon AP, Thomson MA, Harvey P, Valentine A, Davies SE, Walker-Smith JA. (1998). Ileal-lymphoid-nodular hyperplasia, non specific colitis, and pervasive developmental disorder in children. Lancet, 1998; 351 (9103): 637–41. https://doi.org/10.1016/s0140-6736(97)11096-0.
Hyperlink to PDF: https://www.thelancet.com/action/showPdf?pii=S0140-6736%2897%2911096-0.

C. Iversen (✉)
Jefferson Health, Abington, PA, USA
e-mail: Christian.Iversen@jefferson.edu

J. Russell, N. S. Skolnik (eds.), *Top Articles in Primary Care*,
https://doi.org/10.1007/978-3-031-25620-2_58

- No clear association was found between gross gastrointestinal tract examination and histologic samples. Lymphoid nodular hyperplasia was identified in ten patients. Histology showed acute inflammatory changes in five patients and chronic inflammatory changes in eleven patients.
- A temporal association was suggested between MMR vaccination and the onset of behavioral changes and colitis. Behavioral changes were reportedly noted by parents or physicians following measles, mumps, and rubella (MMR) vaccination in eight patients, with average onset 6.3 days following vaccination.

Updates

Around publication, Andrew Wakefield held a press conference thought to have initially fueled the widespread connection between the MMR vaccine and autism. He stated: "there is no proven link as such, and we are seeking to establish whether there is a genuine causal association between the MMR and this syndrome or not. It is our suspicion that there may well be..." and, "I think that [the polyvalent MMR vaccine] should be suspended in favor of the single vaccines" [1]. This association was countered the same year as the title article was published. Results of a 14-year study based in Finland, which followed 1.5 million children, showed no association between a two-dose live-virus (MMR) vaccine and developmental disorders or inflammatory bowel disease [2]. Similarly, in 2001 a retrospective analysis between 1988 and 1993 in the United Kingdom showed a fourfold increase in the diagnosis of autism in boys aged 2–5 years despite stable vaccination rates >95% [3]. This same year, the Medical Research Council (MRC) published a summary report, including numerous international studies, which found no causal relationship between the MMR vaccine and autism [4].

In 2004, investigative journalist Brian Deer released an article in *The Sunday Times* which exposed financial conflicts of interest that Andrew Wakefield failed to disclose to co-authors or *The Lancet* [5].

Soon following this investigation, most authors on the title article called for its retraction, stating: "we wish to make it clear that in this paper no causal link was established between MMR vaccine and autism as the data were insufficient. However, the possibility of such a link was raised and consequent events have had major implications for public health. We consider now is the appropriate time that we should together formally retract the interpretation placed upon these findings in the paper" [6]. From 2007 to 2010, the UK General Medical Council (GMC) conducted hearings into allegations of misconduct by authors Andrew Wakefield, John Walker-Smith, and Simon Murch [7]. In the same period, Brian Deer's investigations demonstrated data manipulation, including falsified symptom and pathology reports [8].

The GMC found Wakefield guilty on numerous counts, including misrepresenting the investigators' roles in patient recruitment causing biased selection; performing invasive testing without clinical indications; misrepresentation (fabrication) of methods and results; failing to disclose professional and financial conflicts of interests; and abusing his authority by obtaining blood samples from children at his child's party. The council found evidence of serious professional misconduct. John Smith and Simon Murch were found not guilty.

Following the GMC investigation and report in 2010, *The Lancet* formally retracted the title paper. The same year, the GMC called for the removal of Andrew Wakefield from the medical register given his "continued lack of insight as to his misconduct" [5].

Importance

Vaccinations are a pillar of preventative medicine. They have reduced the incidence, severity, and complications of numerous illnesses [9], and are attributed to saving an estimated 3 million lives annually worldwide. Importantly, vaccines are also extremely safe. An analysis of the Vaccine Adverse Event Reporting System (VAERS) between 1991 and 2001 showed approximately 18,000 serious adverse events from over 1.9 billion administered doses [10]. Despite their proven benefits and safety, vaccine hesitancy continues to contribute to morbidity and mortality. Studies have linked non-medical exemption to vaccination with numerous outbreaks of measles and pertussis. Although difficult to quantify, the title paper fueled mistrust in the MMR vaccine and contributed to unnecessary harm.

References

1. Deer B. Royal Free MMR video news release. 1998. https://briandeer.com/wakefield/royal-video.htm.
2. Peltola H, et al. No evidence for measles, mumps, and rubella vaccine-associated inflammatory bowel disease or autism in 14-year prospective study. Lancet. 1998;351:1327.
3. Kaye JA, Melero-Montes M, Jick H. Mumps, measles, and rubella vaccine and the incidence of autism recorded by general practitioners: a time trend analysis. BMJ. 2001;322:460–3.
4. MRC Research Council. MRC review of autism research: epidemiology and causes. 2001. https://www.ukri.org/wp-content/uploads/2021/12/MRC-011221-AutismResearchReview.pdf.
5. Deer B. Revealed: MMR research scandal. The Sunday Times. 2004. https://briandeer.com/mmr/lancet-deer-1.htm.
6. Murch SH, et al. Retraction of an interpretation. Lancet. 2004;363(9411):750.
7. General Medical Council. Fitness to practise panel hearing. 2010. https://cdn.factcheck.org/UploadedFiles/gmc-charge-sheet.pdf.
8. Deer B. MMR doctor Andrew Wakefield fixed data on autism. The Sunday times. 2009. http://archive.today/sSQqT.
9. Andre FE, et al. Vaccination greatly reduces disease, disability, death and inequity worldwide. Bull World Health Organ. 2008;86(2):140–6.
10. Zhou W, et al. Surveillance for safety after immunization: vaccine adverse event reporting system (VAERS)—United States, 1991—2001. MMWR. 2003;52(ss01):1–24.

11. Editors of Lancet. Retraction—ileal-lymphoid-nodular hyperplasia, non-specific colitis, and pervasive developmental disorder in children. Lancet. 2010;375(9713):445.
12. Ehreth J. The global value of vaccination. Vaccine. 2003;21(7–8):596–600.
13. Jansen VAA, et al. Measles outbreaks in a population with declining vaccine uptake. Science. 2003;301(5634):804.
14. Phadke VK, et al. Association between vaccine refusal and vaccine-preventable diseases in the United States: a review of measles and pertussis. JAMA. 2016;315(11):1149–58.

Part XII
Pharmacology

John Russell

Chapter 59
Vitamin C and the Prevention of Respiratory Infections-1974

John Russell

Background

Vitamin C stands out among vitamins. Between the time of Columbus and the mid-1800s, it is estimated that 2 million sailors died of scurvy [1]. Vitamin C was the first vitamin synthesized, and the discovery of its synthesis was awarded a Nobel Prize in 1937. The US RDA for vitamin C is only 75–90 mg per day and annual worldwide sales exceed a billion dollars. In a book in 1971, Nobel Laureate Linus Pauling proposed people taking 1–2 g of vitamin C daily and proposed its use for colds. Does that have credence?

Objective

In 1973, a group of Navajo children at a boarding school were evaluated as to whether large doses of vitamin C can impact the development and severity of URIs.

Coulehan JL, Reisinger KS, et al. N Eng J Med. Jan 3, 1974. 290:6 10.
https://www.nejm.org/doi/pdf/10.1056/NEJMoa1107579?articleTools=true.

J. Russell (✉)
Jefferson Health, Abington, PA, USA
e-mail: John.russell@jefferson.edu

J. Russell, N. S. Skolnik (eds.), *Top Articles in Primary Care*,
https://doi.org/10.1007/978-3-031-25620-2_59

Design and Methods

There were 641 Navajo children at a boarding school; over a 14-week period they were randomized to 1 or 2 g of daily vitamin C or placebo. They were followed for the number, type, and length of respiratory illnesses. Students had vitamin C levels assessed.

Results

- The children that received vitamin C had fewer colds and their colds were 30% shorter in duration.
- Those with higher blood levels had shorter illnesses.
- There were more children that had zero illnesses in the vitamin C groups.

Updates

- There was a similar study done in 868 Navajo children in 1976, by the same author, that found no effect of vitamin C on colds [2].
- A Cochrane database from 2013 on vitamin C stated "Regular ingestion of vitamin C had no effect on common cold incidence in the ordinary population, based on 29 trial comparisons involving 11,306 participants. However, regular supplementation had a modest but consistent effect in reducing the duration of common cold symptoms, which is based on 31 study comparisons with 9745 common cold episodes. In five trials with 598 participants exposed to short periods of extreme physical stress (including marathon runners and skiers) vitamin C halved the common cold risk" [3].
- There was interest in the use of intravenous vitamin C in sepsis in the intensive care unit. A study from 2022 showed that it did not help patients on pressor therapy [4].

Bottom Line

There is little evidence that vitamin C helps prevent colds. There may be some better evidence in protecting those that exercise at cold temperatures. Because any excess vitamin C is readily excreted and even if it does little good, at low oral doses it probably does little harm.

References

1. Brown SR. Scurvy. New York, NY: St Marin's Press; 2005.
2. Coulehan JL, Eberhard S, et al. N Engl J Med. 1978;295:73–7.
3. Hemilä H, Chalker E. Vitamin C for preventing and treating the common cold. Cochrane Database Syst Rev. 2013;1.
4. Lamontagne F, Masse MH, et al. Intravenous vitamin C in adult sepsis in intensive care unit. N Engl J Med. 2022;386:2387–239.

Chapter 60
The Porter Letter: The Link between Long-Term Opioids and Addiction-1980

Erin Russell and John Russell

Background

Between 1999 and 2020, more than 564,000 people in the US died from opioid-related overdoses [1]. In 2020, national opioid dispensing rates were 43.3 prescriptions per 100 people; certain areas of the country continue to dispense at disproportionately high rates, with 3.6% of U.S. counties dispensing enough opioid prescriptions for every person in the county to receive one [1]. The national opioid dispensing rate peaked in 2012 with a rate of 81.3 per 100 people. Though prescription rates have decreased to 43.4 prescriptions per 100 people in 2022, opioid-related overdoses continue to remain alarmingly high [1]. Many patients who were started on prescription opioids, who could no longer get these prescriptions from their doctor, bought prescription medications on the street or turned to products like heroin/fentanyl. As of 2022, opioid-related overdose deaths have increased more than eightfold from 1999, with more than 1500 people dying from opioid-related overdoses per week [1, 2]. In conjunction with the COVID-19 pandemic in 2020,

---

Porter, J. (1980). Addiction rare in patients treated with narcotics. New England Journal of Medicine, 302(2), 123–123. https://doi.org/10.1056/nejm198001103020221.
Article PDF: https://www.nejm.org/doi/pdf/10.1056/NEJM198001103020221?articleTools=true.

E. Russell
Temple University School of Medicine, Philadelphia, PA, USA

Jefferson Health, Abington, PA, USA
e-mail: erin.russell@temple.edu

J. Russell (✉)
Family Medicine, Jefferson Health, Philadelphia, PA, USA
e-mail: John.russell@jefferson.edu

J. Russell, N. S. Skolnik (eds.), *Top Articles in Primary Care*,
https://doi.org/10.1007/978-3-031-25620-2_60

the number of opioid-related death rates increased by 38% from 2019 to 2020, especially with the rise in popularity of synthetic opioids such as fentanyl [1]. In 2022, as many as one in four patients on long-term opioid therapy in the primary care setting experiences addiction [1].

Objective

- To determine the rate of opioid addiction in hospitalized patients (without addiction history) who were treated with at least one narcotic preparation in the in-patient setting.

Design and Methods

- Researchers examined files of 39,946 hospitalized patients and monitored closely for opioid addiction.

Results

- Of the 39,946 patients examined, 11,882 were prescribed at least one narcotic preparation, and only 4 of those patients were found to subsequently develop documented addiction.

Importance

In the 5-sentence letter to the editor in 1980, the "Porter Letter" concluded that "despite widespread use of narcotic drugs in hospitals, the development of addiction is rare in medical patients with no history of addiction." Though Porter and Jick only studied hospitalized patients, as the article began to accrue citations, the sentiment that "narcotics are safe and non-addictive" was incorrectly extrapolated and applied to the outpatient setting. In a 2017 analysis of articles that cited the Porter Letter, 72.2% cited the letter as evidence that "addiction was rare in patients treated with opioids" [3]. Importantly, 80.8% of the analyzed citations failed to state that the original Porter study only discussed hospitalized patients, creating a nationally accepted false narrative that opioids were safe and non-addictive in all settings [3]. In a 1998 commercial, the maker of OxyContin, Purdue Pharma, even used the letter to claim that less than 1% of patients treated with opioids become addicted [4].

This sentiment help fuel the U.S. Opioid Epidemic; the introduction of a false narrative was followed by an increase in opioid prescriptions in the 1990s (alongside development of OxyContin in 1995), with prescription rates peaking in 2012 [1, 3]. As now known, opioids can be addictive and dangerous, and unfortunately are still widely used and misused; in 2019, an estimated 10.1 million people aged 12 or older had misused opioids within the past year, with 9.7 million misusing prescription pain relievers [5].

Updates

- In 2007, OxyContin's manufacturer as well as three senior executives pleaded guilty to criminal charges for misleading doctors and the general public about the risk of addiction with opioid use [3].

Bottom Line

- The ongoing U.S. Opioid Epidemic can be traced back to a 5-sentence letter to the editor that briefly discussed how opioids are non-addictive in hospitalized patients. This was a letter, not a validated study. When it was referenced as the "Porter study in the New England Journal of Medicine," doctors were misled to think this was a peer-reviewed study. The findings were largely misinterpreted by academics, many citing the letter as evidence that opioids are non-addictive in all patients in any setting. This false sense of safety led to an increase in opioid prescriptions in the outpatient setting that has fueled the national addiction crisis.

References

1. Centers for Disease Control and Prevention. Prescription opioids. Atlanta, GA: Centers for Disease Control and Prevention; 2017. https://www.cdc.gov/opioids/basics/prescribed.html. Accessed 15 Aug 2022.
2. Council on Foreign Relations. The U.S. opioid epidemic. Council on Foreign Relations. 2022. https://www.cfr.org/backgrounder/us-opioid-epidemic. Accessed 15 Aug 2022.
3. Leung PTM, Macdonald EM, Stanbrook MB, Dhalla IA, Juurlink DN. A 1980 letter on the risk of opioid addiction. N Engl J Med. 2017;376(22):2194–5. https://doi.org/10.1056/nejmc1700150.
4. Health Policy Politics. Purdue pharma OxyContin commercial. *YouTube* YouTube. 2016. https://www.youtube.com/watch?v=Er78Dj5hyeI. Accessed 15 Aug 2022.
5. (DCD), D. C. D. Opioid crisis statistics. HHSgov. 2021. https://www.hhs.gov/opioids/about-the-epidemic/opioid-crisis-statistics/index.html. Accessed 15 Aug 2022.

Chapter 61
Antioxidants and Macular Degeneration-2001

Anne Sprogell

Background

In people aged 65 years or older, age-related macular degeneration (AMD) causes more visual impairment and blindness than any other condition. At the time of publication of this paper, there were a few medical and surgical interventions being studied, but none had been found to be effective. Observational studies have suggested that antioxidants and zinc might slow age-related macular degeneration and the visual impairments it causes.

Objective

This study aimed to "evaluate the effect of high-dose vitamin C and E, beta carotene, and zinc supplements on AMD progression and visual acuity" [1].

A Randomized, Placebo-Controlled, Clinical Trial of High-Dose Supplementation with Vitamins C and E, Beta Carotene, and Zinc for Age Related Macular Degeneration and Vision Loss. (2001). Archives of Ophthalmology, 119(10), 1417. doi: 10.1001/archopht.119.10.1417.
https://www.ncbi.nlm.nih.gov/pmc/articles/PMC1462955/.

A. Sprogell (✉)
Jefferson Health, Abington, PA, USA

J. Russell, N. S. Skolnik (eds.), *Top Articles in Primary Care*,
https://doi.org/10.1007/978-3-031-25620-2_61

Design and Methods

- Double-blind, randomized, controlled trial.
- Participants assigned to 4 arms—placebo, antioxidants (vitamin C, vitamin E, beta carotene), zinc, antioxidants plus zinc.
- Most patients were on a multivitamin of some brand, but the doses of antioxidants were much higher in the trial arm.
- Study measured whether or not patients progressed from Category 1 AMD to higher categories through Category 4 (determined by eye exam findings) and visual acuity.
- Patients were followed for an average of 6 years.

Results

The only findings with statistical significance were that antioxidants plus zinc reduced the progression of disease in patients already in Category 3 and 4 (more advanced AMD) and reduced the loss of visual acuity. There was an increase in progression to AMD and lung cancer for patients in the antioxidant category who smoked, thought to be related to the beta carotene in the antioxidants.

Importance

A follow-up study noted that 8 million adults in the USA fall into the category of people who would benefit from the antioxidant plus zinc supplements. If the AMD of these 8 million people were left untreated, 1.3 million would progress to more advanced AMD and would have decreased visual acuity. If treated with antioxidants and zinc, 300,000 would avoid progression and avoid loss of visual acuity [2].

Bottom Line

The NHANES study from 2017 to 18 showed that 67.3% of patients in the USA over 60 years of age take a dietary supplement. These are often taken with little support for this practice. This study shows a very clear benefit. The article concludes with the recommendation that people 55 years or older should have dilated eye exams and those in Category 3 or 4 of AMD should consider taking a supplement of antioxidants plus zinc. Patients who smoke should avoid beta carotene.

References

1. Age-Related Eye Disease Study Research Group. A randomized, placebo-controlled, clinical trial of high-dose supplementation with vitamins C and E, beta carotene, and zinc for age-related macular degeneration and vision loss. Arch Ophthalmol. 2001;119(10):1417. https://doi.org/10.1001/archopht.119.10.1417.
2. Bressler NM, et al. Potential public health impact of age-related eye disease study results. Arch Ophthalmol. 2003;121(11):1621. https://doi.org/10.1001/archopht.121.11.1621.

Part XIII
Preventive Medicine

Mathew Clark

Chapter 62
Periodic Health Screening-1975

Mathew Clark

Background

At the time this series of articles was written, the idea of critically thinking about periodic, preventive health screening was in its infancy. Academics in Public Health were in the early stages of thinking through, in a systematic way, the questions "What makes a good screening test"? and "Does periodic health screening improve health or decrease morbidity and mortality"? [1] No one in the primary care world had put together an evidence-based list of recommendations for who we should be screening, for what conditions, with what modalities, and how often. Paul Frame and Stephen Carlson were family physicians, associated with the newly minted Family Practice residency programs at the Hunterdon Medical Center in Lambertville, NJ, and the Tri-County program in Dansville, NY. They decided to examine the available evidence and propose a longitudinal screening program for asymptomatic adults.

Frame PS, Carlson SJ. (1975). A critical review of periodic health screening using specific screening criteria Part 1: selected diseases of the respiratory, cardiovascular, and central nervous systems. The Journal of Family Practice, 2(1):29–35. https://www.mdedge.com/familymedicine/issue/182644/journal-family-practice-21

M. Clark (✉)
Jefferson Health, Abington, PA, USA
e-mail: mathew.clark@jefferson.edu

J. Russell, N. S. Skolnik (eds.), *Top Articles in Primary Care*,
https://doi.org/10.1007/978-3-031-25620-2_62

Objective

To produce evidence-based recommendations for periodically screening asymptomatic adults in a primary care setting.

Design and Methods

- The authors propose six criteria to justify screening for a disease or condition:
  - The disease must have a significant effect on quality or quantity of life.
  - Acceptable methods of treatment must be available.
  - The disease must have an asymptomatic period during which detection and treatment significantly reduce morbidity and/or mortality.
  - Treatment in the asymptomatic phase must yield a therapeutic result superior to that obtained by delaying treatment until symptoms appear.
  - Tests must be available at reasonable cost to detect the condition in the asymptomatic period.
  - The incidence of the condition must be sufficient to justify the cost of screening.
- They identified 36 common diseases, which were selected based on their incidence, prevalence, and death rate, using actuarial tables [2], information from the American Cancer Society, and other sources.
- For these selected diseases, available literature was examined, and recommendations were made for screening.
- This paper, the first in a series of four, addressed smoking, HTN, CAD, rheumatic heart disease, Stroke, tuberculosis, lung cancer, brain tumors, and COPD.

Results

- Smoking: Take a smoking history initially, and repeat at ages 30 and 40.
- HTN: Check blood pressure every 2 years.
- CAD: BP every 2 years, cholesterol every 4 years (this was before statins), smoking history every 10 years, weight every 4–6 years. Do not do a screening EKG.
- Rheumatic Heart Disease: Cardiovascular history and physical examination at age 21.
- Stroke: Risk factor screening as for CAD. Interestingly, smoking was not included, as it was not recognized as a stroke risk factor in 1975.
- Tuberculosis: Screen with PPD initially and every 10 years.
- Lung Cancer: No screening recommended (this was pre-CT scan, and screening CXR made no difference in mortality).

- Brain tumors: No screening recommended.
- COPD: Screen for smoking.

Importance

The concept of screening tests needing to meet prespecified criteria presented in this paper is almost taken for granted now. The critical concept that the disease must have an asymptomatic period during which detection and treatment significantly reduce morbidity and/or mortality is a core aspect that many subsequent randomized screening trails have been constructed to prove. While many of the specific recommendations have been superseded by new knowledge and technological advances, the concepts that originated in this paper form the core criteria for screening studies to this day. It is fascinating to read this paper, and to see primary care physicians who are a lot like us, in a new academic discipline, thinking through the available information, and coming up with an evidence-based approach to preventive screening which is still very much relevant almost 50 years later.

Bottom Line

It is possible to take an evidence-based approach to periodic health screening for a variety of common conditions.

References

1. Cochrane AL, Holland WW. Validation of screening procedures. Br Med Bull. 1971;27:3–6.
2. Robbins LC, Geller H. Probability tables of deaths in the next ten years from specific causes. Health hazard appraisal. Indianapolis, IN: Methodist Hospital of Indiana; 1972.

Chapter 63
Fitness and Coronary Artery Disease-2004

Carolyn Sciblo

Background

Many studies have shown the association between overweight or obesity and cardiovascular risk; likewise, many studies have shown the association between physical activity and cardiovascular risk. Women with coronary heart disease (CHD) were excluded from many of those studies, and many of the studies enrolled far more men than women, so the relationship of overweight, obesity, and physical activity in women required more information. This study assessed data from the Women's Ischemia Syndrome Evaluation (WISE) study to evaluate the relationship between physical fitness and obesity measures with heart disease and adverse events.

Objective

- To investigate the relationship among obesity measures (including BMI, waist circumference, waist-hip ratio, and waist-height ratio) and physical fitness (as measured by the self-reported Duke Activity Status Index [DASI]) and degree of physical activity (measured by the Postmenopausal Estrogen-Progestin

Wessel TR, Arant, CB, Olson, MB, et al. Relationship of physical fitness vs body mass index with coronary artery disease and cardiovascular events in women. JAMA, 2004; 292:1179–1187. Hyperlink to article PDF: https://jamanetwork.com/journals/jama/fullarticle/199393.

C. Sciblo (✉)
Temple Health Chestnut Hill Family Medicine, Philadelphia, PA, USA

J. Russell, N. S. Skolnik (eds.), *Top Articles in Primary Care*,
https://doi.org/10.1007/978-3-031-25620-2_63

Intervention questionnaire [PEPI-Q] scores) with coronary artery disease risk factors, angiographic CAD, and adverse cardiovascular events in women who were evaluated for suspected myocardial infarction.

Design and Methods

- Women's Ischemia Syndrome Evaluation (WISE) study enrolled 936 women between 1996 and 2000 with chest discomfort, suspected MI, or both, who were referred for coronary angiography and assessed for adverse outcomes during a mean follow-up of 3.9 years.
- Assessed obesity and fitness via various physical measurements and DASI and PEPI-Q scores; DASI and PEPI-Q scores were correlated with treadmill functional capacity and validated in a WISE cohort sub-study.
- Follow-up data about adverse events was collected 6 weeks after enrollment and then yearly either in person or via telephone.
- Adverse events were defined as all-cause death or hospitalization for nonfatal MI, stroke, congestive heart failure, unstable angina, or other vascular events.

Results

- Cohort was mostly white women who were overweight or obese.
- No difference in presence or severity of angiographic CAD across the BMI categories.
- Lower PEPI-Q and DASI scores were significantly associated with obstructive CAD, but no significant relationship found between body measurements and risk of obstructive CAD.
- DASI and PEPI-Q scores were significantly associated with risk of all adverse events, major events, and all-cause mortality before adjusting for other factors; after adjustment, DASI and PEPI-Q scores were significant predictors of all adverse and major adverse events, but not mortality.
- Women with DASI scores 25 or greater had significantly greater event-free survival than women with scores below 25, regardless of BMI.

Importance

Physical activity as an independent risk factor for cardiovascular events had previously not been validated in a large female cohort. This study illustrated the association between physical activity and heart health in women, separate from weight and other body measurements. This means that focusing solely on weight, and not separately addressing exercise habits and physical fitness, was an inadequate intervention to reduce women's cardiovascular risk. The first female-specific recommendations for preventive cardiology were published in 1999 [1]. In the American Heart Association's 2004 update, "a minimum of 30 minutes of moderate-intensity physical activity on most, and preferably all, days of the week" was a class I recommendation [1]. Women should be counseled both on the importance of maintaining healthy body weight and the benefits of regular physical activity in regard to cardiovascular risk and events.

Updates

In 2007, the American Heart Association (AHA) released another update which retained the above recommendation for 30 min of activity most days of the week as well as included specific activity recommendations for women trying to lose weight or maintain weight loss:

Women should accumulate a minimum of 30 min of moderate-intensity physical activity (eg., brisk walking) on most, and preferably all, days of the week *(Class I, Level B)*.
Women who need to lose weight or sustain weight loss should accumulate a minimum of 60–90 min of moderate-intensity physical activity (e.g., brisk walking) on most, and preferably all, days of the week *(Class I, Level C)* [2].

The 2011 update offered more specifics on the timing and intensity of exercise and incorporating muscle-strengthening exercises as listed below:

Women should be advised to accumulate at least 150 min/week of moderate exercise, 75 min/week of vigorous exercise, or an equivalent combination of moderate- and vigorous-intensity aerobic physical activity. Aerobic activity should be performed in episodes of at least 10 min, preferably spread throughout the week *(Class I; Level of Evidence B)*.
Women should also be advised that additional cardiovascular benefits are provided by increasing moderate-intensity aerobic physical activity to 5 h (300 min)/week, 2½ h/week of vigorous-intensity physical activity, or an equivalent combination of both *(Class I; Level of Evidence B)*.
Women should be advised to engage in muscle-strengthening activities that involve all major muscle groups performed on ≥2 day/week *(Class I; Level of Evidence B)*.
Women who need to lose weight or sustain weight loss should be advised to accumulate a minimum of 60–90 min of at least moderate-intensity physical activity (eg, brisk walking) on most, and preferably all, days of the week *(Class I; Level of Evidence B)* [3].

In 2008, the US Department of Health and Human Services (HHS) published the first *Physical Activity Guidelines for Americans*. In 2018, they released the second edition. They do not include gender-specific guidelines for adults but do agree with the AHA's recommendation for a minimum of 150 minutes of physical activity a week [4].

Bottom Line

- Reported levels of physical fitness among women were better predictors of cardiovascular and all-cause mortality when compared to BMI and other anthropometric measurements. These reported fitness scores had significant associations with cardiovascular events, even after controlling for other cardiovascular risk predictors.

References

1. Mosca L, Appel LJ, Benjamin E, et al. Evidence-based guidelines for cardiovascular disease prevention in women. Circulation. 2004;109:672–93.
2. Mosca L, Banka CL, Benjamin EJ, et al. Evidence-based guidelines for cardiovascular disease prevention in women: 2007 update. Circulation. 2007;115:1481–501.
3. Mosca L, Benjamin EJ, Berra K, et al. Evidence-based guidelines for the prevention of cardiovascular disease in women: 2011 update. Circulation. 2011;123:1243–62.
4. U.S. Department of Health and Human Services. Physical activity guidelines for Americans. 2nd ed. Washington, DC: U.S. Department of Health and Human Services; 2018.

Chapter 64
Smoking and Risk of Lung Cancer: A 50 Year Evaluation-2004

Jonathan P. Andrews

Background

Cigarette smoking steadily became the dominant tobacco product consumed in the United States in the early part of the twentieth century [1, 2]. With this rise in tobacco consumption came increased mortality rates related to lung cancer; however linking the two together did not come until the popularity of cigarettes became well ingrained in society [2]. This study was conceived to evaluate, prospectively, the mortality associated with cigarette smoking when it was at its peak [1, 2].

Objective

- To compare the hazards of cigarette smoking in men who formed their habits at different periods and the extent of the reduction in risk when cigarette smoking is stopped at different ages.

Doll, R., Peto, R., Boreham, J., Sutherland, I. Mortality in relation to smoking: 50 years' observations on male British doctors British Medical Journal. 22 June 2004.
Article PDF: https://www.bmj.com/content/328/7455/1519

J. P. Andrews (✉)
Jefferson Health, Abington, PA, USA
e-mail: Jonathan.Andrews@jefferson.edu

J. Russell, N. S. Skolnik (eds.), *Top Articles in Primary Care*,
https://doi.org/10.1007/978-3-031-25620-2_64

Design and Methods

- Prospective study lasting from 1951 to 2001.
- 34,439 male British physicians were surveyed about their smoking habits from 1951 to 2001 and cause-specific mortality was monitored.
- Main outcome of overall mortality by smoking habit, considering separately men born in different time periods.

Results

- Researchers found the sooner a patient stopped smoking, the sooner their mortality rates declined or improved back to that of non-smoker rates.
- Men who stopped smoking at ages 60, 50, 40, or 30 gained approximately 3, 6, 9, or 10 years of life expectancy.
- The probability of dying middle-aged (35–69) was nearly double to triple the death rates in smokers vs. non-smokers.
- Cigarette smokers die, on average, about 10 years younger than their non-smoker counterparts.

Importance

The public perception of cigarette smoking has drastically changed since the first cigarettes were introduced at the end of the nineteenth century. Today, it is commonplace to see anti-tobacco advertisements on television, radio, and on tobacco products themselves warning about the harmful effects they can cause. What is taken as a matter of fact today, however, was not always the case. During the early part of the twentieth century, cigarettes were viewed by many as a stress relief to combat the horrible realities facing young men fighting in World War I [2]. The tobacco industry capitalized on this unhealthy distraction and was able to firmly cement its place in military, and later civilian, daily life by being included as part of a daily ration provided for by the U.S. government [2]. Following WWI, civilian demand for cigarettes steadily grew, with another major growth spurt following WWII [2].

As our unhealthy consumption for cigarettes grew, so did our understanding of their harmful effects including association with lung cancer, emphysema, and increased mortality, to name a few [1]. This study was initiated in 1951, at the height of the cigarette's popularity, as a prospective cohort analysis to follow over 34,000 men over the course of their lives and determine what effect, if any, smoking cigarettes would have on their mortality. The results the authors have presented are striking and have been instrumental in changing public opinion on cigarette smoking. In addition, this study has very likely contributed to the increase in life expectancy of most Americans from 46 and 48 years (male and female respectively) in 1900 to 76 and 81 in 2016 [4].

2018 saw the fewest number of American adults endorse smoking cigarettes, only 16% of the total population, down from a high of 45% in 1953 [5]. Despite the advances in public awareness, about 250 billion cigarettes were sold in the United States in 2017 alone, and contributed to more than $300 billion in related medical costs in 2016 [3]. Cigarette smoking remains a very prevalent issue affecting many U.S. adults today and is still a major cause for morbidity and mortality. Family physicians are in a great position to provide the necessary, repeated attempts to help patients quit.

Bottom Line

- Cigarette smokers die, on average, about 10 years younger than their non-smoker counterparts.
- Researchers found the sooner a patient stopped smoking, the sooner their mortality rates declined or improved back to that of non-smokers.

References

1. Doll R, Peto R, Boreham J, Sutherland I. Mortality in relation to smoking: 50 years' observations on male British doctors. BMJ. 2004;328(7455):1519.
2. Brandt A. The cigarette century: the rise, fall, and deadly persistence of the product that defined America. Basic Books; 2007.
3. Smoking & Tobacco use: Economic trends in Tobacco. Centers for Disease Control and Prevention. https://www.cdc.gov/tobacco/data_statistics/fact_sheets/economics/econ_facts/index.htm#anchor_1548357749071
4. Life expectancy at birth, at age 65, and at age 75, by sex, race, and hispanic origin: United States, selected years 1900–2016. Centers for Disease Control and Prevention. https://www.cdc.gov/nchs/data/hus/2017/015.pdf
5. Dugan, A. In U.S., smoking rate hits new low at 16%. July 2018. https://news.gallup.com/poll/237908/smoking-rate-hits-new-low.aspx

Part XIV
Pulmonary

Aarisha Shrestha

Chapter 65
Adding LABA to Asthma Therapy (SMART)-2006

Marie Madden

Background

Salmeterol is a long-acting bronchodilator (LABA) that acts by stimulating B2 receptors in the airway smooth muscle. In contrast to Albuterol, which has a 4- to 6-h effect, Salmeterol has a 12-h duration of action. The results of a 1993 RCT comparing the efficacy of Salmeterol vs Albuterol in overall asthma control reflected an overall improvement in asthma control, yet a nonsignificant increase in mortality was shown, in patients assigned to salmeterol.

Objective

This study aimed to further investigate the effect of Salmeterol, when added to baseline asthma treatment, on asthma- and respiratory-related deaths.

Sears, M. R. (2006). The salmeterol multicenter asthma research trial. Chest, 130(3), 928. https://doi.org/10.1378/chest.130.3.928.
https://journal.chestnet.org/article/S0012-3692(15)31518-X/fulltext

M. Madden (✉)
Jefferson Health, Abington, PA, USA

J. Russell, N. S. Skolnik (eds.), *Top Articles in Primary Care*, https://doi.org/10.1007/978-3-031-25620-2_65

Design and Methods

- RCTs of 26,355 subjects with asthma, ages 12 and up, were assigned to either salmeterol or placebo treatment. Both treatment groups continued on their current maintenance medication.
- Four-week follow-ups were performed by telephone call for 28 weeks.
- End points:
  - Primary end points: combined respiratory-related deaths or life-threatening experiences
  - Secondary end points: combined asthma-related deaths or life-threatening experiences, all-cause death, all-cause hospitalization, combined all-cause death of life-threatening experience, respirator-related death, asthma-related death

Results

- The primary end point of combined respiratory-related deaths or life-threatening experiences showed a small, but nonstatistically significant increase in mortality. The relative risk (RR) was 1.33, 95% confidence interval (CI) 0.91–2.14.
- There were statistically significant differences noted in the secondary end points:
  - Asthma-related deaths RR 4.37.
  - Respiratory-related deaths RR 2.16.
  - Combined asthma related deaths or life-threatening episode RR 1.71.
  - The primary end point in African Americans had a RR of 4.10 although the white population has no statistically significant difference in any primary or secondary end points.
- Post hoc analysis showed the use of an inhaled corticosteroid (ICS) at baseline eliminated all the differences seen in the primary and secondary end points in all the populations studied albeit the study was not designed or powered to examine this phenomenon.

Importance

This study provides the evidence behind current guidelines regarding the use of long-acting beta agonists in the treatment of asthma. Whereas the 1993 study highlighted the benefits of Salmeterol on overall asthma control, this study demonstrates an increased mortality rate with the use of Salmeterol when used in the absence of inhaled corticosteroids. Although there is evidence that Salmeterol has a beneficial effect on asthma control, it should not be used alone in the management of asthma. Therefore, current guidelines recommend starting with a short-acting beta agonist and escalating to an inhaled corticosteroid before integrating long-acting beta agonists into maintenance therapy.

Updates

LABA monotherapy has disappeared from the landscape, but the combination of LABA/ICS medications is the cornerstone of both the asthma and COPD guidelines.

Bottom Line

Salmeterol alone for the treatment of asthma leads to increased rate of asthma- and respiratory-related deaths. This increase in mortality is seen specifically in African Americans and those not currently using an inhaled corticosteroid. Salmeterol should be used in combination with inhaled corticosteroids for moderate-persistent asthma.

Chapter 66
Long-acting Beta-agonist Plus Inhaled Corticosteroid in COPD (TORCH)-2007

Jeffrey Matthews

Background

Chronic obstructive pulmonary disease caused an estimated 3.2 million deaths in 2015 [1] accounting for about 5% of global mortality. Before 2007, it was common practice in COPD care to prescribe an inhaled steroid alone such as fluticasone, or a combination inhaled steroid such as fluticasone and a long-active bronchodilator such as salmeterol. The inhaled steroid was used as a way of treating the inflammatory component of the disease and thus reduce exacerbations and mortality. The evidence for utilization of long-acting bronchodilators and inhaled corticosteroids, until the 2007, Towards a Revolution in COPD Health (TORCH) trial, consisted of a retrospective analysis that demonstrated reduced morbidity and mortality with the use of inhaled steroids alone [2] with conflicting meta-analysis of several smaller RCTs showing no reduction in mortality and the ISOLDE study showing that cessation of corticosteroids led to more exacerbations but, unfortunately, did not comment on mortality [3]. At the time, it was still unclear whether corticosteroids alone or in combination with a long-acting bronchodilator would reduce mortality in individuals with COPD. The TORCH trial stands as one of the most robust double-blinded randomized controlled trials to evaluate inhaled corticosteroids with long-acting bronchodilators alone or in combination to reduce morbidity and mortality in COPD.

Calverley, P. M. A., Anderson, J. A., Celli, B., Ferguson, G. T., Jenkins, C., Jone, P. W., … Vestbo, J. (2007). Salmeterol and Fluticasone propionate and survival in chronic obstructive pulmonary disease. The New England Journal of Medicine, 356(8), 775–789. Retrieved from www.nejm.org. Hyperlink to article for our PDF version of the book (will likely handout thumb drives to prospective applicants with our PDF version on it).

J. Matthews (✉)
Jefferson Health, Abington, PA, USA

J. Russell, N. S. Skolnik (eds.), *Top Articles in Primary Care*,
https://doi.org/10.1007/978-3-031-25620-2_66

Objective

To assess whether salmeterol 50 μg and fluticasone 500 μg alone or in combination, used twice per day, would decrease morbidity and mortality in COPD.

Design and Methods

Patients between 40 and 60 years of age, 75% male, diagnosed with COPD with an FEV1 present predicted <60%, with at least a 10 pack year smoking history (both active and non-active smokers), across 444 centers in 42 countries were randomized to either receive placebo, salmeterol 50 μg, fluticasone 500 μg, or a combination of salmeterol 50 μg and fluticasone 500 μg, twice per day over 3 years. The primary end points were death from any cause, post-treatment spirometry, health status evaluated with the St. George's questionnaire (lower scores are better), and exacerbations defined as the need for antibiotics, oral steroids, hospitalization, or a combination of any of the three.

Results

- Mortality in Hazard Ratios and *P* values (some results were omitted; these are the highlights)
  - For all-cause mortality within the 3-year window, combination therapy vs placebo had a favorable hazard ratio of 0.820 with a $P = 0.04$; however the combination therapy vs placebo was not statistically significant adjusted analysis (it is unclear whether the study was powered enough to find statistical significance for mortality benefit or if there is no mortality benefit).
  - Hazard ratio of COPD-related deaths for combination therapy vs. placebo was 0.78 with a nonsignificant *P* value that equals 0.11. In the specific subgroup of COPD death, no benefit in mortality was seen with combination therapy.
  - Combination therapy had a favorable hazard ratio compared to fluticasone in both all-cause mortality and COPD-related death specifically.
- Exacerbations
  - The annual rate of moderate or severe exacerbations had a reduced hazard ratio for all interventions vs placebo. The largest reduction in the ratio of exacerbations was for the combination group vs placebo.

  - For exacerbations requiring hospitalizations, both combination therapy vs placebo and the salmeterol vs placebo had *P* values <0.05 and nearly equivalently reduced hazard ratios 0.83 and 0.82, respectively.
- Pneumonia
  - The authors reported that there was a statistically significant increase in the rate of pneumonia in groups receiving ICS. The probability of reporting pneumonia as an adverse event over the three-year study period was 19.6% in the combo group and 18.3% in the fluticasone-only group as compared to 12.3% and 13.3% in the placebo and salmeterol groups respectively with *P* values <0.001. Over the three-year study period less than 10 people died from pneumonia in each group except for the fluticasone-only group in which 13 people died.

Importance

This large randomized controlled trial established the use of combined inhaled steroid and long-acting bronchodilators for the reduction of exacerbations of COPD. Further, it demonstrated a lack of efficacy with the use of inhaled steroids alone. This trial has been used to set treatment guidelines including the most recent GOLD guidelines and the CHEST guidelines on the treatment of COPD [4].

Updates

Since this trial, the TRILOGY trial has since shown that a long-acting muscarinic antagonist added along with an inhaled corticosteroid and a long-acting bronchodilator was superior to only using a long-acting beta agonist along with an inhaled steroid, as established in the TORCH trial [5]. The SUMMIT trial published in 2016 which looked at fluticasone furoate (ICS) in combination with vilanterol (LABA) vs placebo also failed to demonstrate a statistically significant reduction in mortality. It did not show an increased rate of pneumonia as compared to the TORCH trial.

Bottom Line

The TORCH trial demonstrated evidence for reduced exacerbations with the combined use of Salmeterol and Fluticasone (a LABA and an ICS). It also demonstrated a lack of efficacy and potential harm using inhaled corticosteroids alone in the treatment of COPD.

References

1. Global, regional, and national deaths, prevalence, disability-adjusted life years, and years lived with disability for chronic obstructive pulmonary disease and asthma, 1990–2015: a systematic analysis for the Global Burden of Disease Study 2015.
2. Sin DD, et al. Inhaled corticosteroids and mortality in chronic obstructive pulmonary disease. Thorax. 2005;60(12):992–7. https://doi.org/10.1136/thx.2005.045385.
3. Alsaeedi A, Sin DD, Mcalister FA. The effects of inhaled corticosteroids in chronic obstructive pulmonary disease: a systematic review of randomized placebo-controlled trials. Am J Med. 2002;113(1):59–65. https://doi.org/10.1016/s0002-9343(02)01143-9.
4. Gold reports for personal use—Global Initiative for Chronic Obstructive Lung Disease. (2019). https://goldcopd.org/gold-reports/. Available 10 Nov 2019.
5. Singh D, Papi A, Corradi M, Pavlišová I, Montagna I, Francisco C, et al. Single inhaler triple therapy versus inhaled corticosteroid plus long-acting β2-agonist therapy for chronic obstructive pulmonary disease (TRILOGY): a double-blind, parallel group, randomised controlled trial. Lancet. 2016;388(10048):963–73. https://doi.org/10.1016/s0140-6736(16)31354-X.

Chapter 67
Once-Daily Single-Inhaler Triple vs Dual Thearpy in Patients with COPD-2018

Tricia Cavanaugh

Background

Dual therapy for COPD with either a long-acting anti-muscarinic (LAMA) and a long-acting beta-agonist (LABA) or an inhaled corticosteroid (ICS) and LABA was the mainstay of treatment of COPD. It was uncertain whether there were significant benefits for patients who were prescribed triple therapy with ICS-LAMA-LABA.

Objective

- The Informing the Pathway of COPD Trial (IMPACT) was designed to assess the benefits of triple therapy versus dual therapy with either a LAMA-LABA or ICS-LABA for patients with COPD [1].
- The primary outcome was the annual rate of moderate or severe COPD exacerbations [1].
- Secondary outcomes included improvement in FEV1, time to first moderate or severe exacerbation, time to first exacerbation of any severity in patients with serum eosinophil counts of at least 150 cells/μL, and annual rate of severe exacerbations [1].

Dual therapy with either a long-acting anti-muscarinic (LAMA) plus a long-acting beta-agonist (LABA) or an inhaled corticosteroid (ICS) plus a LAMA has been the mainstay of treatment for COPD.

T. Cavanaugh (✉)
Jefferson Health, Abington, PA, USA
e-mail: Tricia.cavanaugh@jefferson.edu

J. Russell, N. S. Skolnik (eds.), *Top Articles in Primary Care*,
https://doi.org/10.1007/978-3-031-25620-2_67

Design and Methods

- This study was a double-blind, randomized, controlled trial with 10,355 patients with COPD.
- The study was conducted over 52 weeks.
- Patients were at least 40 years old and had symptomatic COPD as defined by COPD Assessment Test (CAT) score >10. They also had either an FEV1 <50% with a history of moderate or severe exacerbations or an FEV1 of 50–80% and at least two moderate or at least one severe exacerbation in the preceding year.
- Baseline chest X-ray was done at the time of the study, and patients would record symptoms daily via an electronic diary. A diagnosis of pneumonia or COPD exacerbation was made by the investigators.
- Patients were maintained on their own medications during a 2-week run-in at the beginning of the trial.
- Study medications used the same ICS, LAMA, and LABA (fluticasone-umeclidinium-vilanterol, umeclidinium-vilanterol, and fluticasone-vilanterol).

Results

- Patients in the triple therapy group had a significantly lower rate of moderate or severe COPD exacerbations compared to either dual therapy. A similar pattern was seen when looking at the rate of all exacerbations.
- Patients in the triple therapy and ICS-LABA groups had lower rates of death from cardiovascular and pulmonary causes.
- Increased rates of pneumonia were seen in the study groups using ICS containing inhalers.
- Improved FEV1 measurements were seen in the triple therapy group.

Importance

This study showed that triple therapy significantly reduced the rates of COPD exacerbations, including moderate and severe exacerbations. The study also demonstrated improvement in lung function in patients using triple therapy. The IMPACT trial showed a decrease in all-cause mortality in patients using triple therapy versus dual therapy options; however, the authors note that this is a fragile finding, which requires further study [1].

Bottom Line

- Triple therapy resulted in a lower rate of moderate or severe COPD exacerbations and hospitalizations than dual therapy in the population selected.

Reference

1. Lipson DA, Barnhart F, Brealey N, et al. Once-daily single-inhaler triple versus dual therapy in patients with COPD. N Engl J Med. 2018;378:1671–80.

Chapter 68
As Needed LABA/ICS in Asthma (START)-2019

Carrie L. Bender

Background

Mild asthma causes a substantial burden with respect to risk of exacerbations [1]. This risk can be reduced with the use of inhaled glucocorticoid therapy [2]. This treatment is often not used due to health care professional reluctance to prescribe and patient reluctance to take it when their symptoms are mild and infrequent [3]. The Novel Symbicort Turbuhaler Asthma Reliever Therapy [Novel START] clinical trial investigates budesonide-formoterol reliever therapy used on an as-needed basis among adults with mild asthma who had been treated with only as-needed SABA.

Objective

To compare budesonide-formoterol use to albuterol use as needed for the prevention of asthma exacerbations.

Beasley, Richard, Holliday, Mark, et al. Controlled trial of budesonide-formoterol as needed for mild asthma. N Engl J Med 2019; 380:21. https://www.nejm.org/doi/full/10.1056/NEJMoa1901963#:~:text=The%20results%20of%20this%20randomized,with%20albuterol%20used%20as%20needed.

C. L. Bender (✉)
Jefferson Health, Abington, PA, USA
e-mail: carrielynn.bender@jefferson.edu

J. Russell, N. S. Skolnik (eds.), *Top Articles in Primary Care*, https://doi.org/10.1007/978-3-031-25620-2_68

Design and Methods

- The study was a 52-week, randomized, open-label, parallel-group, controlled trial involving adults with mild asthma.
- Patients were randomly assigned to one of three groups.
  - albuterol group
  - budesonide plus as-needed albuterol (budesonide maintenance group)
  - budesonide-formoterol group
- Electronic monitoring of inhalers was used to measure medication use.
- Primary outcome was the annualized rate of asthma exacerbations.

Results

- The annualized exacerbation rate in the budesonide-formoterol group was lower than that in the albuterol group and did not differ significantly from the rate in the budesonide maintenance group.
- The number of severe exacerbations was lower in the budesonide-formoterol group than in both the albuterol group and the budesonide maintenance group.
- The incidence and type of adverse events reported were consistent with those in previous trials and with reports in clinical use.

Importance

Prior to the Novel START trial, asthma guidelines recommended ICS for maintenance therapy in patients with more than intermittent asthma (SABA therapy >2 days/week). It allowed patients to use their assigned medications in a more real-world way, without the use of a twice-daily placebo as in previous trials. It also included a subset of those for whom daily steroids are recommended but who were excluded from the two SYGMA trials. This trial was the first to show reduced exacerbation rates as compared with both SABA alone and scheduled ICS plus SABA. The Novel START trial also expanded the indication for intermittent ICS/LABA use to initiation therapy for mild asthma when SABA alone is not enough.

Bottom Line

In an open-label trial involving adults with mild asthma, budesonide-formoterol used as needed was superior to albuterol used as needed for the prevention of asthma exacerbations.

References

1. Dusser D, Montani D, Chanez P, et al. Mild asthma: an expert review on epidemiology, clinical characteristics and treatment recommendations. Allergy. 2007;62:591–604.
2. Reddel HK, Busse WW, Pedersen S, et al. Should recommendations about starting inhaled corticosteroid treatment for mild asthma be based on symptom frequency: a post-hoc efficacy analysis of the START study. Lancet. 2017;389:157–66.
3. Cochrane MG, Bala MV, Downs KE, Mauskopf J, Ben-Joseph RH. Inhaled corticosteroids for asthma therapy: patient compliance, devices, and inhalation technique. Chest. 2000;117:542–50.

Chapter 69
Triple Inhaled Thearpy at Two Glucocorticoid Doses in Moderate-to-Very-Severe COPD-2020

Tricia Cavanaugh

Background

Studies have previously shown the benefits of triple therapy with inhaled corticoste roids (ICS), long-acting muscarinic antagonists (LAMA), and long-acting beta agonists (LABA). However, previous studies only evaluated triple therapy at a fixed inhaled corticosteroid dose, and data showing the impact of other doses of inhaled corticosteroids were lacking.

Objective

- The Efficacy and Safety of Triple Therapy in Obstructive Lung Disease (ETHOS) trial is a stage 3, randomized, controlled trial designed to compare the efficacy and safety of two triple therapy combinations with different doses of ICS compared with dual therapy regimens (LAMA-LABA, ICS-LABA).
- The primary endpoint was the annual rate of moderate or severe COPD exacerbations.
- Secondary outcomes included time to first moderate or severe exacerbation, annual rate of severe exacerbations, change in baseline use of as needed rescue

Hyperlink to PDF.

T. Cavanaugh (✉)
Jefferson Health, Abington, PA, USA
e-mail: Tricia.cavanaugh@jefferson.edu

J. Russell, N. S. Skolnik (eds.), *Top Articles in Primary Care*,
https://doi.org/10.1007/978-3-031-25620-2_69

medication in 24 weeks, percentage of patients who had improvement in St George Respiratory Questionnaire (SGRQ) of more than 4 points in 24 weeks, and time to death from any cause.

Design and Methods

- Stage 3, randomized, double-blind, parallel group trial that was conducted in 26 countries over 52 weeks, and included 8509 patients.
- Patients were at least 40–80 years old and had symptomatic COPD as defined by COPD Assessment Test (CAT) score >10. Patients were receiving at least two inhaled maintenance therapy at the time of selection. They also had an FEV1 <70% with a post-bronchodilator FEV1 of 25–65% of predicted normal value. In the year before screening, patients with an FEV1 <50% had to have a documented history of at least one moderate or severe exacerbation; those with an FEV1 >50% had to have documented at least two moderate or at least one severe exacerbation in the preceding year. They had a smoking history of at least 10 pack years.
- Four different inhaled medication combinations were used; triple therapy with budesonide (either 320 μg or 160 μg), 18 μg glycopyrrolate, and 9.6 μg formoterol; 18 μg glycopyrrolate plus 9.6 μg formoterol; 320 μg budesonide plus 9.6 μg formoterol.

Results

- Patients in both triple therapy groups had a significantly lower rate of moderate or severe COPD exacerbations compared to either dual therapy. No difference was observed between the two triple therapy groups.
- Both triple therapy groups prolonged the time to first exacerbation when compared to either dual therapy group.
- The rate of severe exacerbations was significantly lower in the higher dose triple therapy group when compared to the ICS-LABA group, but not when compared to the LAMA-LABA group. The lower dose triple therapy group showed no difference when compared to either dual therapy group.
- Risk of death was decreased in the higher dose triple therapy group when compared to either dual therapy; the risk of death in the lower dose triple therapy group was lower than the LAMA-LABA group, but higher than the ICS-LABA group.
- Rates of pneumonia were higher in groups containing ICS therapy, and the time to first pneumonia was lower in the LAMA-LABA group when compared to the others.

Importance

The ETHOS trial supports findings from prior studies, including the IMPACT, TRILOGY, and TRIBUTE trials, which show significantly lower rates of moderate to severe COPD exacerbations in patients treated with triple therapy. The data also show improvement in rates of severe COPD exacerbations and patient reported data, such as use of rescue medication and SGRQ response. While the study was not powered to evaluate dose-response between the triple therapy groups, the trends in the data were similar, and interestingly the lower dose triple therapy group, which contained 160 μg of budesonide, showed superiority over the ICS-LABA, which contained 320 μg of budesonide.

Bottom Line

- At both standard and low ICS doses, the triple-combination therapy showed a statistically significant reduction in the rate of moderate or severe exacerbations compared with dual-combination therapies.

Further Reading

Rabe KF, Martinez FJ, Ferguson GT, Wang C, Singh D, Wedzicha JA, et al. ETHOS investigators. Triple inhaled therapy at two glucocorticoid doses in moderate-to-very-severe COPD. N Engl J Med. 2020;383:35–48.

Part XV
Women's Health

Amy Clouse

Chapter 70
Introduction of Combined Hormonal Oral Contraceptives-1958

Amy Clouse

Background

Prior to the twentieth century, contraception generally consisted of abstinence, breast feeding, withdrawal methods, and animal gut condoms. Margaret Sanger (founder of the precursor to Planned Parenthood) and Katharine McCormick (a wealthy socialite) were instrumental in supporting the initial clinical trials of a contraceptive pill [1]. This pill, Enovid©, developed from the work of Dr. Gregory Pincus, was initially approved by the Federal Drug Administration (FDA) in 1957 as treatment for menstrual disorders [1]. This is one of the first published clinical trials of Enovid© for fertility control that led to additional FDA approval as a contraceptive method in March of 1960.

Objective

- The objective of this study was to prove the contraceptive effectiveness of an oral combination of a synthetic progesterone, norethynodrel, and an estrogen, the 3-methyl ether of ethinyl estradiol, mestranol.

Pincus G, Rock J, Garcia CR et al. Fertility control with oral medication. American Journal of Obstetrics and Gynecology 1958;75: 1333–1346. PMID: 13545267 DOI: 10.1016/0002-9378(58)90722-1.
Hyperlink to PDF: https://www.ajog.org/article/0002-9378(58)90722-1/pdf.

A. Clouse (✉)
Jefferson Health, Abington, PA, USA
e-mail: amy.clouse@jefferson.edu

J. Russell, N. S. Skolnik (eds.), *Top Articles in Primary Care*,
https://doi.org/10.1007/978-3-031-25620-2_70

Design and Methods

- This was considered a field trial of a combination of a synthetic progesterone and estrogen pill. There was no placebo group.
- The subjects were 265 married women living in a low-income housing development in Puerto Rico. Their median age was 27.4 and they were followed for 16 months.
- The study drug contained 10 mg of norethynodrel, an oral progestational agent (that had already been shown in animals and a select group of humans to suppress ovulation), and varying amounts of the drug, ethinyl estradiol 3-methyl ether, mestranol. Women were instructed to take the tablet on days 5 through 24 of their menstrual cycle.
- Compliance with the study medication was monitored by a trained social worker who visited women in their homes at each medication cycle for pill counts, to deliver the next cycle's tablets and to monitor side effects, length of menstrual cycle, frequency of coitus, and number of missed tablets.
- Some participants also came to the office and had pelvic examinations, endometrial biopsies, blood work and urine samples for steroid levels.

Results

- Adequate data was available for a total of 1712 menstrual cycles for the 265 women. Of these, 1279 were reported with no medication omissions, 282 with one to five missed tablets and 151 with 6–19 missed tablets.
- In those women with no missed tablets, cycle lengths were consistent at approximately 27 days. Cycle lengths became less consistent with more missed tablets.
- There were no pregnancies in the group with no missed pills, indicating 100% efficacy. In the group who had missed one to five tablets, there were 2 pregnancies and in the group with six or more missed pills, there were 3 pregnancies.
- There were also 14 pregnancies in women who had stopped the medication due to side effects. This total of 19 pregnancies in the study indicates an overall pregnancy rate of 13 per 100 marriage years (now called woman years), compared to an expected 67 per marriage years in those not using contraception, according to the authors who cited unpublished comparative data.
- Side effects included breast tenderness, nausea, vomiting, and pelvic pain in up to 27% of participants. The authors compared the incidence of side effects in this study to their previous studies of only the progestin component and noted that side effects were more frequent when estrogen was present. They also indicated that side effects were highest in the first cycle of the study medication and were lower in later cycles.

Importance

This study and other related work from Dr. Pincus helped Enovid© garner FDA approval as the first oral contraceptive pill in 1960.

Updates

- Soon after FDA approval, Enovid© use increased rapidly in the United States. However thrombotic events were noted and by 1963, the FDA had over 350 reports of thromboembolic events and 12 deaths [2]. Enovid© did contain a relatively high amount of estrogen compared to modern-day combined contraceptive pills. (For comparison, the estrogen dose in the original pill was equivalent to about 100 μg of ethinyl estradiol whereas our current combined oral contraceptive pills usually contain between 10 and 35 μg of ethinyl estradiol.) Since that time, it has been removed from the market and doses of ethinyl estradiol in oral contraceptive pills have progressively been lowered to avoid thrombotic events
- In addition to combined oral contraceptive pills, there are other non-oral delivery routes for estrogen and progestin combination contraception such as the vaginal ring and transdermal delivery systems. Furthermore, there are numerous other options now available for contraception, both hormonal and not, including progestin only pills, injectable progestins, and the long-acting reversible contraceptives such as progestin implants and progestin and copper intrauterine devices.

Bottom Line

According to United Nations data in 2019, 151 million women use combined oral contraceptive pills worldwide, accounting for 16% of all contraception users [3]. While adverse effects and dosing had yet to be determined, this early work was pivotal in understanding ovulation suppression and ultimately putting women in control of their own fertility.

References

1. Christin-Maitre S. History of oral contraceptive drugs and their use worldwide. Best Pract Res Clin Endocrinol Metab. 2013;27(1):3–12.
2. FDA Report on Enovid. Ad Hoc advisory committee for the evaluation of a possible etiologic relation with thromboembolic conditions. JAMA. 1963,185(10):776.
3. United Nations, Department of Economic and Social Affairs, Population Division. Contraceptive Use by Method: Data Booklet (ST/ESA/SEA.A/435). New York: United Nations, 2019.

Chapter 71
Folic Acid to Reduce Neural Tube Defects-1992

Anne Sprogell

Background

In Hungary, the country on which this study was focused, the prevalence of isolated neural tube defects was 2.8 per 1000 births. Prior to this study, there was evidence that use of a multivitamin in the periconceptional period prevented recurrent neural tube defects. However, in 95% of cases of neural tube defects, previous children from that family did not have a defect.

Objective

While there was evidence that vitamin supplementation, specifically folic acid, prevented recurrent neural tube defects, this trial aimed to study if vitamin supplementation could reduce the incidence of neural tube defects for all pregnancies, not just in women who had a prior pregnancy with a neural tube defect.

Czeizel, A. E., & Dudás, I. (1992). Prevention of the First Occurrence of Neural-Tube Defects by Periconceptional Vitamin Supplementation. New England Journal of Medicine, 327(26), 1832–1835. doi: 10.1056/nejm199212243272602.
PDF Link: https://www.nejm.org/doi/pdf/10.1056/NEJM199212243272602?articleTools=true.

A. Sprogell (✉)
Jefferson Health, Abington, PA, USA

J. Russell, N. S. Skolnik (eds.), *Top Articles in Primary Care*,
https://doi.org/10.1007/978-3-031-25620-2_71

Design and Methods

- Randomized controlled trial.
- One arm was given a multivitamin containing vitamin A, vitamin B1, vitamin B2, vitamin B6, vitamin B12, vitamin C, vitamin D, vitamin E, calcium pantothenate, biotin, folic acid, calcium, phosphorus, magnesium, iron, copper, manganese, and zinc.
- Second arm given a trace element supplement containing copper, manganese, zinc, and vitamin C.
- Women were provided with multivitamin or trace element supplement 1 month before trying to conceive through the third month of pregnancy, then data was collected on their pregnancies.
- The definition of neural tube defects in this study included anencephaly, iniencephaly, encephalocele, spina bifida cystica, and their combinations and secondary consequences. It did not include spinal dysraphism or spina bifida due to issues diagnosing these conditions in the perinatal period.

Results

- No cases of neural tube defects in 2014 pregnancies in the multivitamin group compared with 6 cases in 2052 pregnancies in the trace element supplement group (p value of 0.029).
- The prevalence of congenital malformations (including neural tube defects) in the multivitamin group was 13.3 per 1000 births compared with 22.9 per 1000 births in the trace element supplement group (p value of 0.02).

Importance

Because of this study and studies that followed, folic acid at 0.4 mg a day is recommended for all women of childbearing age. Because most of the studies provided multivitamins for at least a month before conception, the formation of neural tube defects takes place in the first month when some women don't know they are pregnant, and half of pregnancies in the US are unplanned, it is recommended that even women who aren't planning on becoming pregnant get 0.4 mg of folic acid a day. According to the CDC, after these studies and folic acid recommendations, the FDA began requiring that folic acid be added to grain products labeled as "enriched" in 1998.

Bottom Line

Due to the results from this study and following studies, recommendations on folic acid for women of childbearing age changed. In addition, in a sweeping public health effort, folic acid is now added to any cereal grain product in the US labeled "enriched."

Further Reading

Czeizel AE, Dudás I. Prevention of the first occurrence of neural-tube defects by periconceptional vitamin supplementation. N Engl J Med. 1992;327(26):1832–5.

Women and Folic Acid. 2019. https://www.cdc.gov/ncbddd/folicacid/recommendations.html.

Chapter 72
AZT Treatment to Prevent Maternal-Infant Transmission of HIV-1994

Bhasha Mukhopadhyay

Background

Maternal-infant transmission of Human Immunodeficiency Virus (HIV) type 1 is the primary way babies acquire HIV. In the early years of the HIV epidemic, up to 40% of babies born to HIV positive mothers became infected in utero, during labor and delivery, or by breast-feeding and pediatric HIV was considered a fatal disease, despite treatment. This randomized controlled trial tested a Zidovudine regimen for reducing the risk of maternal-fetal HIV transmission.

Objective

- To test the efficacy of a Zidovudine regimen consisting of antepartum, intrapartum, and postnatal (for infant) dosages in prevention of maternal-fetal HIV transmission.

Connor, E. M., Sperling, R. S., Gelber, R., Kiselev, P., Scott, G., O'Sullivan, M. J., VanDyke, R., Bey, M., Shearer, W., Jacobson, R. L., Jimenez, E., & O'Neill, E. (1994). Reduction of Maternal-Infant Transmission of Human Immunodeficiency Virus Type 1 with Zidovudine Treatment. New England Journal of Medicine, 331, 1173–1180. https://doi.org/10.1056/NEJM199411033311801.
Hyperlink to PDF: https://www.nejm.org/doi/10.1056/NEJM199411033311801?url_ver=Z39.88-2003&rfr_id=ori:rid:crossref.org&rfr_dat=cr_pub%20%200www.ncbi.nlm.nih.gov.

B. Mukhopadhyay (✉)
Jefferson Health Abington, Abington, PA, USA
e-mail: bhasha.mukhopadhyay@jefferson.edu

J. Russell, N. S. Skolnik (eds.), *Top Articles in Primary Care*,
https://doi.org/10.1007/978-3-031-25620-2_72

Design and Methods

- This study was a double-blind, placebo-controlled, randomized study, enrolling pregnant, HIV infected women between 14 and 34 weeks' gestation, with CD4+ T lymphocyte counts >200 cells/mm. 477 pregnant women enrolled at 59 centers between April 1991 and December 1993.
- Women all met the following inclusion criteria: hemoglobin ≥8 g/dL, absolute neutrophil count ≥1000 cells/mm, platelet count ≥100,000 cells/mm, serum ALT ≤2.5 times the upper limit of normal, serum creatinine ≤1.5 mg/dL or 8-h urinary creatinine clearance >70 mL/min.
- Women were excluded if their prenatal ultrasound showed any life-threatening fetal anomaly, oligohydramnios in second trimester or unexplained polyhydramnios in third trimester, fetal hydrops, ascites, or other evidence of fetal anemia. They were also excluded from the study if they had received any antiretroviral therapy, anti-HIV vaccines, cytolytic chemotherapeutic agents, or radiation therapy during this pregnancy.
- In the medication group, Zidovudine was dosed at 100 mg PO 5 times a day in the antepartum period and then 2 mg/kg of body weight IV over 1 h then 1 mg/kg/h until delivery in the intrapartum period. Newborns were given 2 mg/kg PO Q6H for 6 weeks.
- Women were monitored every 4 weeks until 32 weeks' gestation, weekly until delivery, at 6 weeks postpartum and then again at 6 months postpartum. An ultrasound was obtained before entry into the study and then every 4 weeks after the 28th week of gestation. A non-stress test was performed every week starting at gestational age 34 weeks.
- Infants were evaluated at birth and at weeks 1, 2/3, 6, 12, 24, 36, 60, 72, 78 of life.
- Treatment was discontinued if the mother developed severe pre-eclampsia, disseminated intravascular coagulation, recurrent thrombocytopenia, life-threatening or recurrent severe toxic effects, progressive HIV disease requiring treatment with open-label Zidovudine, fetal death, or any of the following lab abnormalities: absolute neutrophil count <750 cells/mm, hemoglobin <8 g/dL, platelet count <50,000 cells/mm· or ALT concentration >5 times the upper limit of age-adjusted normal value.
- Treatment was discontinued in the infant if they had any of the discontinuation criteria above for the mother, any severe toxic effects, or had received an experimental anti-HIV vaccine or drug.
- Infants had peripheral-blood mononuclear cells obtained for HIV culture at birth, week 12 of life, week 78 of life; HIV serologic testing (enzyme immunoassay and Western blot assay) at weeks 72 and 78 of life; later stages of the study also included additional culture at week 24 of life.

Results

- Of the 477 women enrolled in this study, 409 gave birth during the study resulting in 415 live born infants. Women received the study drug for a median of 11 weeks before giving birth.
- At 18 months post-partum, the estimated proportion of infants infected with HIV was 8.3% in the zidovudine group and 25.5% in the placebo group, both with a 95% confidence interval. This corresponded to a 67.5% relative reduction in the risk of maternal-fetal transmission.
- Minimal short-term toxic effects were observed in mothers; only a few women in either the treatment or the placebo group discontinued therapy in the study because of toxic effects.
- For infants, the only short-term toxic effect found was a mild and reversible anemia.

Importance

This was the first study to show that treating mothers with HIV and their infants with a regimen of antepartum, intrapartum, and postnatal Zidovudine is safe and effective in preventing maternal-infant HIV transmission.

Updates

Additional research into combination antiretroviral therapy has now shown that a combined antiretroviral regimen can achieve a risk of 1–2% or less for maternal-to-child transmission if maternal viral loads of 1000 copies/mL or less can be sustained, independent of the route of delivery or duration or ruptured membranes before delivery [1]. Because this is such a significant reduction in transmission rates, the American College of Obstetricians and Gynecologists [2], the American Academy of Pediatrics [3], and the Centers for Disease Control and Prevention (CDC) [4] all recommend an opt-out HIV screening strategy for pregnant women.

Bottom Line

Treating HIV-infected pregnant women with antiretroviral therapy in the antepartum and intrapartum periods and then the infant postnatally is critical for prevention of maternal-fetal HIV transmission. Screening for HIV therefore is very important for primary care providers to remember in those patients planning pregnancy or those that could already be pregnant.

References

1. ACOG Committee Opinion No. 751. American College of Obstetricians and Gynecologists. Labor and delivery management of women with human immunodeficiency virus infection. Obstet Gynecol. 2018;132:e131–7.
2. ACOG Committee Opinion No. 752. American College of Obstetricians and Gynecologists. Prenatal and perinatal human immunodeficiency virus testing. Obstet Gynecol. 2018;132:e138–42.
3. American Academy of Pediatrics, American College of Obstetricians and Gynecologists. Joint statement of ACOG/AAP on human immunodeficiency virus screening. College statement of policy. Washington, DC: AAP, ACOG; 1999.
4. Branson BM, Handsfield HH, Lampe MA, Janssen RS, Taylor AW, Lyss SB, et al. Revised recommendations for HIV testing of adults, adolescents, and pregnant women in health care settings. Centers for Disease Control and Prevention (CDC). MMWR Recomm Rep. 2006;55:1–17.

Chapter 73
Coronary Heart Disease and HRT (HERS Trial)-1998

Kathleen E. Leary

Background

In the late 1980s and early 1990s, numerous observational studies noted lower rates of coronary heart disease (CHD) in women taking postmenopausal estrogen compared to women not taking postmenopausal hormone therapy. This association was noted to be strongest in women with established CHD. The Heart and Estrogen/progestin Replacement Study (HERS) Research Group attempted to answer whether there was a causal relationship between postmenopausal hormone therapy and risk of CHD.

Objective

To see if treatment with estrogen plus progestin affected risk of coronary heart disease (CHD) events in postmenopausal females with known coronary disease.

Hulley, S., Grady, D., & Bush, T. (1998). Randomized Trial of Estrogen Plus Progestin for Secondary Prevention of Coronary Heart Disease in Postmenopausal Women. JAMA, 280(7), 605–613. doi: 10.1001/jama.280.7.605.
Hyperlink to PDF: https://jamanetwork.com/journals/jama/fullarticle/187879.

K. E. Leary (✉)
Jefferson Health, Abington, PA, USA
e-mail: kathleen.leary@jefferson.edu

J. Russell, N. S. Skolnik (eds.), *Top Articles in Primary Care*,
https://doi.org/10.1007/978-3-031-25620-2_73

Design and Methods

- The study was a randomized, blinded, placebo-controlled secondary prevention trial.
- 2763 postmenopausal women, younger than 80 years old, with established coronary disease and an intact uterus participated in the trial. 1380 women were assigned to the treatment arm and 1383 to the placebo arm.
- Age range was 44–79 years old; mean age was 66.7 years. 89% of participants were white.
- Women were randomized to receive a daily dose of 0.625 mg of conjugated equine estrogen plus 2.5 mg of medroxyprogesterone acetate or placebo.
- Women were followed for an average of 4.1 years.
- The primary outcomes were nonfatal myocardial infarction (MI) or CHD death.
- Secondary cardiovascular outcomes included coronary artery bypass graft surgery, percutaneous coronary intervention, admission for unstable angina, resuscitated cardiac arrest, congestive heart failure, stroke, transient ischemic attack, and peripheral arterial disease. Non-cardiovascular secondary outcomes included total mortality, cancer, deep vein thrombosis (DVT), pulmonary embolism (PE), fracture, and gallbladder disease.
- Women who developed endometrial hyperplasia without atypia that did not respond to treatment with progestin, endometrial hyperplasia with atypia, cancer of the endometrium, cervix, breast, or ovary, DVT, PE, gallbladder disease or who required prolonged immobilization were taken off treatment but continued to be followed.

Results

- The primary outcomes of nonfatal MI and CHD death occurred in 172 women in the hormone group and in 176 women in the placebo group. These differences were not statistically significant.
- There was, however, a statistically significant time trend, with more CHD events in the hormone group in year 1 compared to the placebo group and fewer CHD events in year 4 and 5 compared to placebo group.
- Lipid panels were favorably changed in the hormone group, with a net 11% reduction in LDL cholesterol level and 0% increase in HDL cholesterol level in the hormone group compared to the placebo group.
- Women in the hormone group experienced higher rates of venous thromboembolic events (Relative Hazard 2.89) and gallbladder disease (RH 1.38).
- Power was limited for other secondary outcomes, including fracture, cancer, and total mortality. No significant differences were found between hormone and placebo group.

Importance

HERS was the first prospective randomized controlled trial (RCT) to study the impact of menopausal hormone therapy on cardiovascular disease. Not only did it fail to demonstrate the expected outcome of cardiovascular protection based on results of observational studies, in fact it showed increased risk of harm among the treated group. Broadly, HERS underscores the fact that RCTs are needed to evaluate the risks and benefits of therapies, no matter how strong observational evidence appears.

Updates

Subsequent to HERS, two large trials from the Women's Health Initiative were published in 2002 and 2004. These trials, looking at conjugated equine estrogen alone in women with hysterectomy [1] as well as estrogen plus progestin [2], were both stopped early after noting a number of adverse outcomes among the treatment group, including increased risk of stroke, coronary heart disease, venous thromboembolism, and breast cancer. In 2017, the United States Preventative Services Task Force (USPSTF) did a meta-analysis of 18 trials looking at menopausal hormone therapy. Based on these results, the USPSTF recommended "against the use of combined estrogen and progestin [as well as the use of estrogen alone] for the primary prevention of chronic conditions in postmenopausal women. (D recommendation)" [3].

In the years following these studies, use of menopausal hormone therapy declined precipitously, from a prevalence of 22.4% in 1999–2000 to 4.7% in 2010 [4].

One significant critique of HERS and the WHI studies was that the mean age of women was 66.7 years in HERS and 63 years in WHI. It is important to note that the risk of menopausal hormone therapy for women aged 50–59 was more favorable than for older women.

Bottom Line

Menopausal hormone therapy is no longer recommended for primary prevention of CHD.

References

1. Anderson GL, Limacher M, Assaf AR, Bassford T, Beresford SA, Black H, et al. Effects of conjugated equine estrogen in postmenopausal women with hysterectomy: the women's health initiative randomized controlled trial. JAMA. 2004;291(14):1701–12.
2. Rossouw JE, Anderson GL, Prentice RL, LaCroix AZ, Kooperberg C, Stefanick ML, et al. Risks and benefits of estrogen plus progestin in healthy postmenopausal women: principal results from the women's health initiative randomized controlled trial. JAMA. 2002;288(3):321–33.
3. US Preventive Services Task Force. Hormone therapy for the primary prevention of chronic conditions in postmenopausal women: US preventive services task force recommendation statement. JAMA. 2017;318(22):2224–33. https://doi.org/10.1001/jama.2017.18261.
4. Sprague BL, Trentham-Dietz A, Cronin KA. A sustained decline in postmenopausal hormone use: results from the National Health and Nutrition Examination Survey, 1999-2010. Obstet Gynecol. 2012;120(3):595–603. https://doi.org/10.1097/AOG.0b013e318265df42. PMID: 22914469; PMCID: PMC3607288.

Chapter 74
Endometrial Sampling Accuracy 2000

Morgan Katz

Background

There are multiple methods for assessing endometrial cells for cancer and hyperplasia including biopsy or sampling, dilation and curettage (D&C), and hysteroscopy. An invasive D&C was the method of choice for many years; however studies had questioned its accuracy as less than half of the uterine cavity is curetted in the majority of cases. Assessment of abnormal uterine bleeding with endometrial biopsy or sampling of cells is a less invasive technique compared to D&C or hysteroscopy. This chapter aimed to perform meta-analysis of prior studies to determine the accuracy of endometrial sampling to detect endometrial carcinoma and atypical hyperplasia in the diagnostic workup of abnormal bleeding.

Objective

- To perform a meta-analysis of multiple studies to determine the accuracy of endometrial sampling compared to more invasive methods.

Dijkhuizen, F. P., Mol, B. W., Brölmann, H. A., & Heintz, A. P. (2000). The accuracy of endometrial sampling in the diagnosis of patients with endometrial carcinoma and hyperplasia: a meta-analysis. Cancer, 89(8), 1765–1772.
Hyperlink to PDF: https://acsjournals.onlinelibrary.wiley.com/doi/10.1002/1097-0142(20001015)89:8%3C1765::AID-CNCR17%3E3.0.CO;2-F.

M. Katz (✉)
Jefferson Health, Abington, PA, USA

Primary Care, ChristianaCare, Newark, USA

J. Russell, N. S. Skolnik (eds.), *Top Articles in Primary Care*,
https://doi.org/10.1007/978-3-031-25620-2_74

Design and Methods

- The authors performed a literature search for studies published between 1966 and 1999 comparing results of endometrial sampling with findings at D&C, hysteroscopy, and/or hysterectomy.
- They found 39 studies involving 7914 women which were included in the meta-analysis.
- For each study, the authors calculated the fraction of patients in which endometrial sampling failed, and in which endometrial sampling was successful or not successful in diagnosing endometrial carcinoma and atypical hyperplasia.
- This data was then used to determine sensitivity and specificity of endometrial sampling with a variety of devices.

Results

- Detection rate of endometrial carcinoma with endometrial sampling was higher in postmenopausal women compared to premenopausal women.
- The Pipelle device had the highest detection rate of endometrial carcinoma in pre- and post-menopausal women with a sensitivity of 99.6% in post-menopausal women and 91% in pre-menopausal women.
- For detection of atypical hyperplasia, the Pipelle was also found to be the most sensitive technique, with a sensitivity of 81%.
- The specificity of all devices for endometrial sampling was 98%.

Importance

This meta-analysis highlighted the important role of endometrial sampling for the diagnoses of endometrial cancer and hyperplasia. Sampling the endometrium with a Pipelle is both sensitive and specific and provides a less invasive, less expensive alternative to the more traditional D&C and hysteroscopy.

Updates

- Additional meta-analysis published in 2016 in the *European Journal of Obstetrics and Gynecology and Reproductive Biology* showed that the sensitivity of endometrial sampling to detect endometrial cancer may be lower than previously thought. Endometrial sampling is still recommended in the workup of abnormal uterine bleeding, but further workup may be indicated after a benign result of endometrial sampling in a post-menopausal woman.

Bottom Line

Abnormal uterine bleeding is a common complaint and must be worked-up thoroughly to rule out cancer. The American Academy of Family Physicians, the American College of Obstetricians and Gynecologists, and the American Cancer Society all recommend endometrial sampling for patients with abnormal uterine bleeding, especially in post-menopausal women. Endometrial sampling with a Pipelle is an accurate, minimally invasive diagnostic tool that can be performed in a provider's office as part of that workup.

Further Reading

Lei J, Ploner A, Elfström M, Wang J, Roth A, Fang F, Sundström K, Dillner J, Sparén P. HPV vaccination and the risk of cervical cancer. N Engl J Med. 2020;383:1340–8. https://doi.org/10.1056/NEJMoa1917338.

Chapter 75
HPV-16 Vaccine-2002

Dyllan Walter

Background

The sexually transmitted infection Human Papilloma Virus 16 (HPV-16) is known to be a potent carcinogen as it is the most common HPV type associated with cancers of the cervix, anus, and vulva. *Persistent* HPV-16 infection is particularly linked to cervical cancer and dysplasias among women. Early animal studies and human safety and immunogenicity studies using an HPV-16 L1-virus-like particle showed promise in protecting women from persistent HPV-16 infection.

Objective

- The purpose of this study was to evaluate the efficacy of an HPV-16 vaccine in preventing persistent HPV-16 infection in young women.

Koutsky, L.A., Ault, K.A., Wheeler, C.M., Brown, D.R., Barr, E., Alvarez, F.B., Chiacchierini, L.M., & Jansen, K.U. (2002). A controlled trial of a human papillomavirus type 16 vaccine. The New England Journal of Medicine, 347(21), 1645–1651. DOI 10.1056/NEJMoa020586.
Hyperlink to PDF: https://www.nejm.org/doi/full/10.1056/NEJMoa020586.

D. Walter (✉)
Jefferson Health, Abington, PA, USA
e-mail: dyllan.walter@jefferson.edu

J. Russell, N. S. Skolnik (eds.), *Top Articles in Primary Care*,
https://doi.org/10.1007/978-3-031-25620-2_75

Design and Methods

- The researchers conducted a double blind, randomized controlled, multicenter clinical trial of 2392 women, ages 16–23, recruited from 16 locations in and around United States college campuses.
- To be included, women had to have five or fewer male sex partners, no history of abnormal pap smears, and could not be currently pregnant.
- Women were randomized to receive either the study HPV-16 vaccine or the placebo, containing only the adjuvant.
- Vaccines were given at 0, 2, and 6 months in both the study and placebo groups and women documented adverse effects for 2 weeks after each vaccine. Participants were asked again about adverse effects at 2, 6, and 7 months.
- HPV-16 testing via pap smear and vaginal swabs as well as blood testing for HPV-16 antibodies was performed when enrolled, 1 month after the third vaccine, and then every 6 months thereafter for 4 years. The post-vaccine follow-up tests also included HPV DNA testing that did not influence management.
- Those with precancerous abnormalities on pap tests underwent colposcopy and were referred for biopsy if they had abnormal colposcopic findings.
- Investigators analyzed the efficacy of the vaccine among women who received all 3 doses of the study vaccine and conformed to study protocol. They also looked at the efficacy among women who received the vaccine under "a general violation of protocol" which may reflect results from ordinary use.

Results

- Among the 2392 women, those who received study vaccine ($n = 1194$) and placebo ($n = 1198$) were equally represented in the analysis and 64% of those women met criteria for primary analysis. HPV-16 infection at enrollment was the most common reason for women to be excluded from the primary analysis.
- Serum HPV-16 antibodies were significantly higher in women who received 3 doses of the HPV vaccine (mean titer of 1510 mMu/mL) vs the placebo (<6 mMu/mL) with a Confidence Interval (CI) 95%.
- NONE of the women in the study vaccine group developed persistent HPV-16 infection whereas the incidence in the placebo group was 3.8 per 100 women-years at risk (CI 95%, $p < 0.001$).
- The placebo group yielded 41 persistent HPV-16 infections, 5 of which were HPV-16 related CIN-1 and 4 were HPV-16 related CIN-2. Thirty-one were without cervical dysplasia. One did not complete the study.

- A secondary analysis of women who did not perfectly conform to study protocol which could be compared to usual conditions also showed 100% study vaccine efficacy in preventing *persistent* HPV-16.
- The study group did not report significantly more adverse effects than the placebo group; however more women in the study group did not complete the series suggesting it may have been less tolerated. No serious vaccine-related events occurred.

Importance

This study showed that the HPV-16 vaccine prevented persistent HPV infection among women and laid the groundwork for future HPV vaccine studies and our current HPV vaccine recommendations. For ethical reasons, early studies such as this one did not measure cancer as an end point. However, recent data from a large study showed the powerful effects of the HPV vaccine in reducing the incidence of HPV-related cancers [1].

Updates

- The HPV vaccines have evolved since early studies to provide more coverage of high-risk HPV types.
- The first HPV vaccine that was recommended for girls in 2006 by the Advisory Committee on Immunization Practices (ACIP) in the United States was Gardasil© (HPV-4) which included types 6, 11, 16, 18.
- In addition to Gardasil©, Cervarix© became available in 2009 which included types 16 and 18. At that time, ACIP expanded the recommendation to include boys as well.
- HPV-9 vaccine is currently recommended by the ACIP. Because it covers 9 types of HPV (16, 18, 6, 11, 31, 33, 45, 52, 58), it has the potential to prevent the majority of cervical cancers across the world [2].
- Testing for presence of high-risk HPV is now incorporated into cervical cancer screening guidelines and the management algorithms for abnormal pap smears [3].

Bottom Line

- This early study investigated the efficacy of HPV-16 vaccine in preventing persistent HPV-16 infection. It also posited that by preventing HPV, we could reduce the risk of cervical cancer and recent data has supported that assumption. As a safe and effective public health tool, the HPV vaccine continues to be recommended for the prevention of HPV-related cancers, most commonly cervical cancer. It is key that primary care providers share the importance of the HPV vaccine with parents, adolescents, and young adults and dispel common myths about its safety and efficacy.

References

1. Lei J, Ploner A, Elfström M, Wang J, Roth A, Fang F, Sundström K, Dillner J, Sparén P. HPV vaccination and the risk of cervical cancer. N Engl J Med. 2020;383:1340–8. https://doi.org/10.1056/NEJMoa1917338.
2. Markowitz LE, Schiller JT. Human papillomavirus vaccines. J Infect Dis. 2021;224(S4):S367. https://doi.org/10.1093/infdis/iaa621.
3. Perkins RB, Guido RS, Castle PE, Chelmow D, Einstein MH, Garcia F, Huh WK, Kim JJ, Moscicki A, Nayar R, Saraiya M, Sawaya GF, Wentzensen N, Schiffman M. 2019 ASCCP risk-based management consensus guidelines for abnormal cervical cancer screening tests and cancer precursors. J Low Genit Tract Dis. 2020;24(2):102–31. https://doi.org/10.1097/LGT.0000000000000525.

Chapter 76
Risks and Benefits of Estrogen/Progestin in Healthy Women (WHI)-2002

Aarisha Shrestha

Background

Between 1990 and 1992, various research pointed to potential cardio-protection in postmenopausal women users of hormone therapy (HT). Due to the favorable effects of HT on lipids, attention was focused on the possible use of postmenopausal HT as a strategy for primary prevention of cardiovascular disease. 1998's Heart and Estrogen/progestin Replacement Study (HERS) trial reported an apparent increased risk of Coronary Heart Disease (CHD) in the first year of hormone use for those with documented prior CHD [1]. This prompted speculation that any early adverse effect of hormones on CHD incidence was confined to women with prior CHD events. The Women's Health Initiative (WHI) clinical trial looked specifically at this issue of potential risks and benefits of HT for otherwise healthy postmenopausal women. The Women's Health Initiative is a large long-term national health study sponsored by the National Heart, Lung and Blood Institute, focused on preventing heart disease and breast and colorectal cancers. The original study had 3 parts: a clinical trial of postmenopausal hormone use, vitamin D and calcium supplementation and low-fat dietary patterns, an observational trial, and a community prevention

---

Rossouw JE, et al. Risks and benefits of estrogen plus progestin in healthy postmenopausal women: Principal results from the Women's Health Initiative randomized controlled trial. JAMA 2002; 288:321–333.
Hyperlink to PDF: https://jamanetwork.com/journals/jama/fullarticle/195120.

A. Shrestha (✉)
Jefferson Health, Abington, PA, USA
e-mail: Aarisha.shrestha@jefferson.edu

J. Russell, N. S. Skolnik (eds.), *Top Articles in Primary Care*,
https://doi.org/10.1007/978-3-031-25620-2_76

study. The postmenopausal hormone trial had two separate studies: the estrogen-plus-progestin study of women with a uterus and the estrogen-alone study of women without a uterus. This is a review of the most often cited WHI data, the estrogen-plus-progestin combined hormone clinical trial.

Objective

- This part of the WHI clinical trial was designed to assess the risks and benefits of HT with the primary outcome designated as CHD in predominantly healthy women with an intact uterus.
- Secondary outcomes included stroke, venous thromboembolism (VTE), cancer, and osteoporosis.

Design and Methods

- Randomized controlled trial of 16,608 women with an intact uterus.
- Mean participant age of 63 (range 50–79 years).
- The test group received 1 tablet containing conjugated equine estrogen 0.625 mg and medroxyprogesterone 2.5 mg (Prempro).
- Formal monitoring began in 1997 with goals of an average 8.5 years follow-up.

Results

- The study was stopped early after 5.2 years due to evidence of breast cancer harm (26% increase), nominal statistically significant increase in CHD, and statistically significant increase in stroke and VTE. These risks outweighed the benefit of osteoporotic fracture prevention and possible colon cancer prevention.
- Increased risks for CVD and invasive breast cancer were present among women with an increased intact uterus across racial/ethnic and age strata and were not influenced by the antecedent risk status or prior disease. All-cause mortality was not affected during the trial.
- The WHI estrogen-alone study continued for an additional 1.5 years and showed no benefit of estrogen therapy in the prevention of CHD. Those results were reported separately [2].

Table 76.1 Recommendations for hormone replacement

AHA (2011) [5]	Menopausal HT and SERMs should not be used for the primary or secondary prevention of CVD (*Class III*, Level of Evidence A)
USPSTF (2017) [6]	Recommends against the use of combined HT for the primary prevention of chronic conditions in postmenopausal women (grade D)
AAFP [7]	Supports the USPSTF recommendation
ACOG (2013) [8]	Menopausal HT should not be used for the primary or secondary prevention of coronary heart disease at the present time
NAMS (2017) [9]	For women who initiate HT more than 10 or 20 years from menopause onset or are aged 60 years or older, the benefit-risk ratio appears less favorable because of the greater absolute risks of coronary heart disease, stroke, venous thromboembolism, and dementia

Importance

In 2001, the American Heart Association recommended against initiating postmenopausal hormones for the secondary prevention of cardiovascular disease but did not make a firm recommendation for primary prevention [3]. The WHI trial was designed to address this very issue and when published in 2002, it was the first randomized study to show that HT does not confer benefit for preventing CHD among women with an intact uterus. Since then, several guideline-issuing bodies discourage against HT use for primary prevention of CHD (Table 76.1). Since the publication of WHI findings, use of menopausal HT has declined from 44% in 1988–1994 to 4.7% in 2010 [3].

Updates

- WHI revisited the topic in 2013 [10] and found that although HT reduces LDL-C levels, it does not reduce the LDL particle numbers, suggesting that LDL particles may be smaller and more atherogenic overall.
- The Early versus Late Intervention Trial with Estradiol (ELITE) showed that the effect of HT on CVD risk may differ based on early vs late initiation with respect to menopause onset (known as the "Timing Hypothesis"). This trial concluded that when HT is initiated at the time of menopause or within 6 years after menopause, there is a significant reduction in CVD relative to no effect when initiated >10 years after menopause [11]. Thus, some organizations have taken this into account for their recommendations.

Bottom Line

- WHI's randomized controlled trial of estrogen plus progestin in postmenopausal women with an intact uterus showed that postmenopausal hormone therapy should not be initiated or continued for primary prevention of coronary heart disease due to increased risk of CAD, non-fatal MI, invasive breast cancer, stroke, and VTE.

References

1. Hulley S, Grady D, Bush T. Randomized trial of estrogen plus progestin for secondary prevention of coronary heart disease in postmenopausal women. JAMA. 1998;280(7):605–13. https://doi.org/10.1001/jama.280.7.605.
2. Anderson GL, Limacher M, Assaf AR, et al. Effects of conjugated equine estrogen in postmenopausal women with hysterectomy: the Women's Health Initiative randomized controlled trial. JAMA. 2004;291(14):1701–12. https://doi.org/10.1001/jama.291.14.1701.
3. Mosca L, Collins P, Herrington DM, Mendelsohn ME, Pasternak RC, Robertson RM, et al. Hormone replacement therapy and cardiovascular disease. Circulation. 2001;104:499–503.
4. Gartlehner G, Patel S, Viswanathan M, et al. Hormone therapy for the primary prevention of chronic conditions in postmenopausal women: an evidence review for the US preventive services task force: evidence synthesis no. 155. Rockville, MD: Agency for Healthcare Research and Quality. AHRQ Publication; 2017. 15-05227-EF-1.
5. Mosca L, Benjamin EJ, Berra K, Bezanson JL, Dolor RJ, Lloyd-Jones DM, et al. Effectiveness-based guidelines for the prevention of cardiovascular disease in women—2011 update: a guideline from the American Heart Association. Circulation. 2011;123(11):1243–62. https://doi.org/10.1161/CIR.0b013e31820faaf8.
6. US Preventive Services Task Force. Hormone therapy for the primary prevention of chronic conditions in postmenopausal women. US Preventive Services Task Force Recommendation Statement. JAMA. 2017;318(22):2224–33.
7. American Academy of Family Physicians. Clinical preventive service recommendation: hormone replacement therapy. http://www.aafp.org/patient-care/clinical-recommendations/all/hrt.html.
8. American College of Obstetricians and Gynecologists. ACOG Committee Opinion No. 565. Hormone therapy and heart disease. Obstet Gynecol. 2013;121(6):1407–10.
9. NAMS. Hormone therapy position statement advisory panel. The 2017 hormone therapy position statement of the North American Menopause Society. Menopause. 2017;24(7):728–53.
10. Howard BV, Rossouw JE. Estrogens and cardiovascular disease risk revisited: the Women's Health Initiative. Curr Opin Lipidol. 2013;24:493–9.
11. Howard N, Hodis MD, Wendy J, et al. Vascular effects of early versus late postmenopausal treatment with estradiol. N Engl J Med. 2016;374:1221–31. https://doi.org/10.1056/NEJMoa1505241.

Index

J. Russell, N. S. Skolnik (eds.), *Top Articles in Primary Care*,
https://doi.org/10.1007/978-3-031-25620-2

L

M

N

O

P

Q

R

MIX
Papier aus verantwortungsvollen Quellen
Paper from responsible sources
FSC® C105338
FSC
www.fsc.org

If you have any concerns about our products,
you can contact us on
ProductSafety@springernature.com

In case Publisher is established outside the EU,
the EU authorized representative is:
Springer Nature Customer Service Center GmbH
Europaplatz 3, 69115 Heidelberg, Germany

Printed by Libri Plureos GmbH
in Hamburg, Germany